PARASITOLOGY

This accessible reference provides a comprehensive overview of parasitic organisms, covering their practical applications and fundamental concepts that impact global health and ecosystems. From intricate life cycles to advanced diagnostic techniques, the text illuminates the complex world of parasites through clear explanations and visual learning aids. Designed for students and professionals across continents, it serves as an essential resource for infectious disease and public health practitioners. The book's balanced approach to theory and application makes parasitology accessible to readers at various expertise levels while maintaining scientific rigour and clinical relevance.

KEY FEATURES

- Includes pictorial representations that transform complex parasitological concepts into easily digestible visual frameworks.
- Provides chapter-specific resource directories that guide readers towards specialized information sources and relevant professional networks.
- Addresses the critical intersection of parasitology with public health initiatives, conservation efforts, and food security challenges across diverse global contexts.

PARASITOLOGY
An Illustrated Outline

Patrick Ferdinand Ayeh-Kumi

CRC Press
Taylor & Francis Group
Boca Raton London New York

CRC Press is an imprint of the
Taylor & Francis Group, an **informa** business

Designed cover image: Shutterstock

First edition published 2027
by CRC Press
2385 NW Executive Center Drive, Suite 320, Boca Raton FL 33431

and by CRC Press
4 Park Square, Milton Park, Abingdon, Oxon, OX14 4RN

CRC Press is an imprint of Taylor & Francis Group, LLC

ISBN: 9781041227861 (hbk)
ISBN: 9781041223986 (pbk)
ISBN: 9781003733935 (ebk)

DOI: 10.1201/9781003733935

Typeset in Helvetica
by Deanta Global Publishing Services, Chennai, India

This book is dedicated to Professors Samuel Ntow Afuakwa, A. W. Chinnery, Reginald Kwaku Anteson, Mercy Jemima Newman, Julius Addo Mingle, and Kingsley Twum-Danso with deep gratitude and to my wife Lady Beatrice and our boys Ernest, Emmanuel, Ferdinand, and Charles and my dear mother Grace-Beauty Ohenewa Bekoe and all my siblings. I am forever grateful.

Contents

Foreword

It is a distinct honour to contribute this Foreword for the publication of this substantive and timely textbook on parasitology. In an increasingly complex and interconnected world, the discipline of parasitology occupies a critical position at the intersection of human and animal health, environmental stewardship, and global disease management. The appearance of this book is therefore both opportune and essential, offering rigorously presented knowledge and lucid explanations that will serve a wide audience within the biomedical sciences academic space.

The author's scholarly depth and evident commitment to the field are manifested throughout the text. Complex subject matter is articulated with clarity, precision, and pedagogical sensitivity, rendering the material accessible without compromising academic rigour. The systematic organization of the chapters, together with the inclusion of carefully designed diagrams and illustrations, significantly enhances comprehension and supports learners across varying levels of training, particularly undergraduate medical students.

This work extends well beyond the conventional confines of parasitology. While firmly grounded in the foundational principles of the discipline, it also integrates contemporary advancements in molecular biology, immunology, and related biomedical sciences – domains that continue to refine our understanding of parasitic diseases, host–parasite interactions, and emerging pathogenic threats. By weaving together classical concepts with modern scientific developments, the text equips readers with both the conceptual grounding and the analytical tools required to address evolving challenges within the field.

Notably, the book reframes parasitology as a dynamic, intellectually rigorous, and indispensable discipline within modern medical science. It presents a balanced and comprehensive perspective that underscores not only the scientific complexity of parasitic organisms but also the practical relevance of parasitology in clinical, public health, and research contexts.

I am confident that this textbook will serve as an enduring resource for students, educators, researchers, and health professionals. It represents a commendable scholarly contribution and one that I am pleased to recommend with the utmost confidence.

—Professor Mercy Jemima Newman

Preface

Parasitology occupies a vital position within the medical sciences, offering indispensable insights into the biology, pathology, and epidemiology of organisms that affect human health. For undergraduate health sciences students, a sound understanding of parasitic diseases is essential – not only for scientific and clinical competence but also for contributing meaningfully to public health initiatives and research.

The discipline is currently undergoing a significant transformation, driven by advances in molecular biology and immunology. These developments are reshaping traditional paradigms and enhancing our understanding of host–parasite interactions at the cellular and molecular levels. As such, the study of parasitology is evolving from its classical foundations towards a more integrative and mechanistic approach.

This textbook adopts a pragmatic and accessible framework for exploring clinical parasitology. Recognizing that the subject is often perceived as overly technical and abstract, the content has been carefully structured to support progressive learning. Beginning with foundational principles, each chapter builds upon the previous, guiding the reader towards a comprehensive and clinically relevant understanding of parasitic diseases.

To facilitate ease of comprehension, the text is enriched with clear diagrams and illustrations, making complex concepts more approachable for students at varying levels of academic preparation. Topics covered include parasite morphology and classification, life cycles, physiology, immunology, epidemiology, clinical manifestations, diagnostic techniques, and pharmacokinetics of antiparasitic agents.

This book is intended to serve as both an academic resource and a practical guide. It aims to demystify parasitology, foster analytical thinking, and equip future medical professionals and biomedical scientists with the knowledge required to diagnose, manage, and prevent parasitic infections effectively.

It is my hope that this work will inspire curiosity, deepen understanding, and support the academic and professional development of all who engage with it.

—Patrick Ferdinand Ayeh-Kumi

Acknowledgements

I am profoundly indebted to the numerous individuals whose contributions have significantly informed and enriched this edition. Foremost, I acknowledge with deep respect my late mentor and supervisor, Professor Reginald Kwaku Anteson, whose distinguished scholarship and exemplary tutelage cultivated in me a rigorous and enduring foundation in medical parasitology. May his memory remain a blessing and his soul rest in eternal peace.

I am deeply grateful to Professors Constantine Tempelis and Don Heineman (University of California, Berkeley), as well as Professors William Arthur Petri, Moses Kwamena Woode, Richard Littleton Guerrant, and Barbara Mann (University of Virginia, Charlottesville). Their invaluable guidance during my postgraduate studies at both UCB and UVA provided me with essential clarity, direction, and motivation. Their contributions have left an indelible imprint on my professional development.

I am equally grateful to Professor Mercy Jemima Newman, former Head of the Department of Medical Microbiology, and to all past and current Heads of the Department of Medical Microbiology, University of Ghana Medical School. Their sustained encouragement, institutional support, and scholarly leadership played an indispensable role in the successful realization of this book.

My sincere appreciation is extended to Professor Julius Addo Mingle, whose guidance during my formative years in the Department of Medical Microbiology provided clarity, direction, and motivation. His contributions have left an indelible imprint on my professional development.

I further express my gratitude to Professor Kingsley Twum-Danso and Dr. Elizabeth Bannerman for their unwavering support and academic assistance, both of which have been invaluable over the years.

To a daughter, sister, and colleague – Professor Patience B. Tetteh-Quarcoo – I extend profound appreciation for her sustained commitment, intellectual engagement, and steadfast support throughout the development of this work.

My thanks also go to Mr. Addo Osafo Kantanka, Mr. Israel Attipoe, and Mr. Ernest Arthur for their consistent and dedicated technical assistance, which has greatly facilitated the production of this edition.

Special acknowledgement is due to the illustrators whose meticulous and aesthetically refined graphical contributions substantially enhanced the pedagogical value of this text. I am also grateful to colleagues and friends whose constructive critiques and scholarly insights informed the refinement of the manuscript. To the students of the College of Health Sciences, University of Ghana, whose inquiries and feedback reaffirmed the relevance and necessity of this resource, I remain sincerely appreciative.

I further record my gratitude to Isabella Aryee, Peter Baddoo, James Teye Ocansey, Michael Kofi Ottoboah, Divine Ndeogo, and Belinda Deckor, whose diligence, continued commitment, and perseverance – often through numerous revisions and late-night work sessions – were instrumental in ensuring the timely completion of this edition.

Finally, I extend my deepest appreciation to my wife, Beatrice, and to our sons – Ernest, Emmanuel, Charles, and Ferdinand – for their steadfast understanding, encouragement, and support. Their patience and unwavering commitment provided the foundation upon which this scholarly work was completed.

About the Author

Reverend Professor Patrick Ferdinand Ayeh-Kumi is a distinguished professor, renowned medical parasitologist, microbiologist, and laboratory scientist, holding esteemed credentials from the University of Ghana.

Prof. Ayeh-Kumi has a rich academic history. He is a past Provost of the College of Health Sciences of the University of Ghana. Prior to his provostship appointment, he served as the Head of Microbiology, University of Ghana Medical School, and Head of the Department of Medical Laboratory Sciences, School of Allied Health Sciences, University of Ghana. By virtue of hard work and excellence in leadership, he was appointed as Dean of the School of Allied Health Sciences, Dean of the School of Biomedical and Allied Health Sciences, and Acting Dean of the School of Public Health of the University of Ghana.

With an illustrious academic journey, Prof. Ayeh-Kumi earned the distinction of being the first to achieve a PhD in Microbiology from the University of Ghana. He undertook part of his postgraduate studies at the University of California, Berkeley, United States; University of Virginia, Charlottesville, United States; University of Copenhagen, Denmark; and the Galilee College in Israel. He is a Foundation Fellow of the West African Postgraduate College of Medical Laboratory Science (WAPCMLS).

Proficient in his craft, Prof. Ayeh-Kumi's passion extends beyond academia. With over 30 years of dedicated teaching, mentoring, and research, he has left an indelible mark in the field of medical parasitology, microbiology, and biomedical laboratory sciences.

Beyond academia, Prof. Ayeh-Kumi's contributions extend to numerous local and international boards and committees. He is an ordained Minister of the Adonai International Fellowship Alliance Incorporated, Sacramento, California, United States. Prof. Ayeh-Kumi embodies a blend of academic excellence and spiritual dedication. He has been married to Lady Beatrice for 35 years, and they are blessed with four sons.

1 Fundamentals of Parasitology

Great works are performed not by strength but by perseverance.

Samuel Johnson

CHAPTER OUTLINE

In this introductory chapter, you will be introduced to the fundamentals of parasitic organisms and their interactions with hosts. Get ready to embark on a journey where you will:

- *Explore Medical Parasitology*: You will be introduced to the scope and significance of medical parasitology in diagnosing, managing, and preventing diseases caused by various parasites, including arthropods, protozoa, and helminths.
- *Uncover Historical Perspectives*: You will understand the evolution of concepts regarding infectious diseases, from primitive beliefs to modern scientific understanding, highlighting key figures and discoveries that shaped our understanding of parasitic infections.
- *Understand the Concept of Multiple Causation of Diseases*: You will see how interactions between the agent, host, and environment contribute to the occurrence and outcome of parasitic infections.
- *Dive into Host–Parasite Interactions*: You will explore the intricate relationships between parasites and their hosts, including types of symbiotic associations and the diverse influences parasites exert on host organisms.
- *Discover Characteristics of Parasites*: You will uncover the unique biological and physiological adaptations of parasites, including reproductive strategies, anatomical modifications, and life history complexities.
- *Learn about Types of Parasites*: Understanding classification of parasites based on their location, dependence on hosts, and modes of transmission, from ectoparasites to opportunistic parasites.
- *Explore Influences of Parasites on Hosts*: You will see the various ways parasites affect host organisms, from mechanical disturbances and interference with metabolism to production of toxic substances and promotion of secondary infections.

DOI: 10.1201/9781003733935-1

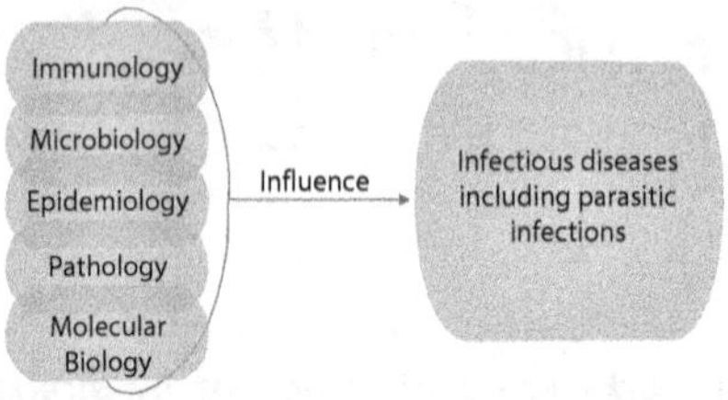

Figure 1.1 Biological disciplines that influence the study of parasites.

1.1 MEDICAL PARASITOLOGY AS A SUBJECT

Medical parasitology is a specialty of medical science concerned with the epidemiology, clinical manifestations, pathology, diagnosis, management, prevention, control, and treatment of illnesses caused by parasites including pathogenic arthropods, protozoa, and (metazoan) helminths. Parasitology takes its roots from zoological sciences but is to a significant extent hinged on other disciplines such as Microbiology, Immunology, Pathology, and Molecular Biology (Figure 1.1).

Recent advances in these related disciplines have given a clear indication that different parasitic agents can utilize similar mechanisms to infect, invade, produce disease, and evade the immune systems of the host. Excluding bacteria, fungi, viruses, and rickettsia, which are technically parasitic in nature, "true" parasitic organisms are still leading in abundance. Host immune/defence strategies and mechanisms elicited against diverse types of parasitic/infectious disease agents may differ, overlap, or could also be quite similar, depending on the status of the agent, i.e., whether the agent is extracellular or intracellular, exogenous or endogenous. Aside from parasites, there are other infectious disease-causing agents; these are listed below.

1.2 TYPES OF INFECTIVE AGENTS

Bacteria	*Fungi*	*Protozoa*	*Viruses*	*Mycoplasma*
Spirochetes	Rickettsia	Viroids	Prions	Helminthes

With the invention of the microscope in the 16th century, one can observe these infective agents of diseases. Anton van Leeuwenhoek (1632–1723), a Dutch draper and cloth merchant, was the first to observe bacteria, yeast, and protozoa. He observed numerous other organisms in water and made detailed drawings of some of these microorganisms.

1.3 HISTORICAL PERSPECTIVE OF THE CHANGING CONCEPTS OF INFECTIOUS (BACTERIAL, PARASITIC, AND VIRAL) DISEASES

1. ***Primitive/supernatural concepts***

   "*Demonology*": In this concept, the belief is that plagues and pestilences are caused or instigated by demons; insinuating a worldview where supernatural entities are responsible for the spread of disease and calamity among humans.

   "*Deity*": Suggests that diseases occur because of the visitation of a displeased God to punish humans/subjects for their sins. Both belong to the supernatural theory and infer that diseases are caused by factors from without and not from within. Primitive concepts also include a lack of scientific understanding, assumptions, and misunderstanding.

2. ***Ancient concepts***

   These concepts thrive on the notion that religion dominated the lives of people. Both illness and healing were therefore considered to be related to the supernatural.

   Ancient Hebrews also believed that disease was related to both "dirt and impurity" and led them to develop programmes in personal hygiene and **sanitation**.

3. ***Greek medicine***

   Hippocrates (460–355 BCE), the father of medicine, discarded the supernatural theory. He believed, as did previous scholars, that the universe consisted of four elements – **air, water, earth, and fire,** and had four opposing elementary properties – **hot/cold and moist/dry**.

   He expounded the humoral theory of disease, which stated that the body had four humours – blood, phlegm, yellow bile, and black bile. When in balance, health prevailed and when out of balance, disease occurred.

   He also observed the seasonal occurrence of respiratory and intestinal diseases and of malaria and related these to the weather/climatic conditions.

4. ***Roman influence***
   Galen (130–200 CE) also discarded the supernatural theory of disease. He did some animal dissections and physiological experiments but was most noted for the philosophy of disease that he set forth; much of it, though wrong, dominated the thinking about the cause of disease for centuries to come. His basic teleology was "that the environment does nothing in vain."

   Environmental sanitation and personal hygiene were important contributions of the Romans.
5. ***Medieval concepts***
   This era brought about the idea of contagious diseases and quarantine. Since there was limited understanding about the spread of diseases, the church attributed diseases to divine retribution for leading a sinful life.
6. ***The Renaissance***
   Girolamo Fracastoro (1493–1541), a scientist from Verona, was the first to study contagion and to present the concept that "**disease is not caused by mysterious shadows or miasmas, nor by obstructed humours, but by a kind of seed – a minute, invisible substance**." He also defined some of the essential characteristics of diseases that are recognized for infectious disease today. Some of these are as follows.

   Three methods of spread:

   - Directly, from a distance and by fomites, disease was transmitted.
   - Transmitted agent propagated itself.
   - Agents show specificity for each disease.

   Anton von Leeuwenhoek (1632–1723) was a Dutch draper by trade who made pioneering contributions to microbiology and microscopy during the Golden Age of Dutch science and technology. Though self-taught and without formal scientific training, he crafted high-powered single-lens microscopes that allowed him to be among the first to observe and describe microorganisms, which he called "animalcules." His work laid the foundations for microbiology as a scientific discipline.
7. ***18th century***
   Edward Jenner (1749–1823) was an English doctor who discovered the smallpox vaccine. In 1800, he vaccinated James Phipps with cowpox material, which resulted in the development of resistance to smallpox infection and thereby established the use of vaccination as a method of infectious disease prevention.

   Theory of spontaneous generation: Holds the belief that living organisms could arise spontaneously from non-living matter. Macro and microorganisms arose spontaneously from decaying meat. Thus, diseases were caused by "spontaneous generation" or by "miasma from decayed matter."

8. ***Modern concepts***

1820: Deodorants were used to reduce putrefaction. Sodium hypochlorite was used in Parisian morgues to reduce decay.

Ignaz Semmelweis was a Hungarian physician who was working in Vienna supervising medical students in the maternity wards when he noted a correlation between putrefaction in autopsy and puerperal fever in pregnant women. During 1840 and 1848, he noticed that some physicians found higher rates of puerperal fever in their patients. He, along with Oliver Wendell Holmes in the US, requested that all of the physicians wash their hands between patients. Few complied, and many more women died in childbirth.

Louis Pasteur disproved the theory of spontaneous generation and together with others, notably Koch, proved the concept that disease was caused by microorganisms. Pasteur, a very bright chemist and brewer of German beer, in 1850 while trying to make the best beer in France, noticed that it was microorganisms that fermented sugar to alcohol. He discovered the existence of anaerobic life. When "incorrect" microbes were in the mixture, undesirable products resulted. He demonstrated the importance of pasteurization and sterilization by heating. He proceeded to culture *Bacillus anthracis* and proved it a causative agent of the disease anthrax.

John Tyndall, when trying to test Pasteur's experiments, discovered the existence of two forms of bacteria: *Heat labile* and *heat resistant* forms. He validated Pasteur's theory and proved that repeated heating (Tyndallization) successfully sterilizes solutions.

Joseph Lister was an English surgeon who introduced the antiseptic principles. Using data gathered in operating rooms and from old bandages he picked up in the waste bins outside hospitals, he proposed that infections were due to "substances" found around patients. He began to use carbolic acid (phenol) to wrap wounds and to spray the air around the patient, which killed what he called "septic germs." His work went unappreciated for years.

Robert Koch (1890) was a German physician who continued Louis Pasteur's work. He established the aetiology of infectious diseases. He established that anthrax bacteria were always present in the infected blood, that the infected blood could transmit anthrax, and the bacteria could be isolated outside the animal. In 1890 he discovered the causative organisms for tuberculosis and cholera.

Koch's Postulates

1. Infectious organisms should be present in hosts with the disease and absent from those without the disease.
2. Infectious organisms must be grown in pure culture in vitro.
3. Inoculation of healthy hosts with pure culture.
4. Resolution of infectious organisms (identical to original isolates) from infected/disease hosts.

Paul Ehrlich's work from 1880 to 1910 established the basis of modern chemotherapy. He used an arsenic-containing compound (salvarsan) to treat syphilis. He and a Japanese expert, Sa Hachiro Hata, developed the antimicrobial drug "magic bullets" using salvarsan and neosalvarsan.

John Snow formulated the theory of communicable diseases during a cholera epidemic in London in 1854. He proposed that each communicable disease had a distinct and specific cause and a causal agent that was a stable living organism. He understood that infection was necessary for disease transmission. He also theorized that the quantity of the infectious material increased through multiplication after infection leading to disease manifestation. His other works include advocating for the use of chloroform as an anaesthetic during surgery.

William Hallock Park proved the concept of carriers of disease. His extensive work on diphtheria helped him discover that those who recovered from the disease still harboured the bacterium in their throats. This caused these "carriers" to be able to transmit the disease to others. He also demonstrated that asymptomatic carriers played a crucial role in disease spread.

Theobald Smith was a pioneering American epidemiologist, bacteriologist, pathologist, and professor. He was one of the earliest researchers to demonstrate transmission of disease by animal vectors.

Many researchers advanced the concept, first demonstrated by John Snow's ingenious studies, that disease was transmitted by contamination of water, soil, air, food, etc.

Spenserian thinking of the "survival of the fittest" has dominated our approach to infectious diseases, even up to today.

Alexander Fleming was a Scottish bacteriologist who discovered penicillin and used it to cure various diseases. He observed that *Penicillium notatum* could kill *Staphylococcus aureus*. He discovered the antibiotic property of penicillin. Along with **Ernst Chain** and **Howard Florey's work in 1940**, he developed a production process.

Joshua Lederberg, Edward Tatum, and George Beadle in 1950 established the basis of heredity and genetic control. They discovered and worked on genetic recombination in bacteria.

Francois Jacob and Jacques Monod (1960) discovered and elucidated control of enzyme synthesis. They are credited with the Lac Operon model of genetic control of enzyme synthesis. They both proposed the existence of an RNA messenger. They found that the balance between regulator and structural genes enables cells to adapt to varying conditions. An interruption in this balance can stimulate the production of new enzymes, which may benefit or harm the cell.

Michael Bishop and Harold Varmus in 1980 discovered that virus-encoded oncogenes originate in eukaryotic cells. Their findings revealed how malignant tumours form due to changes in normal cell genes, shedding light on the mechanisms underlying cancer development.

Kary Mullis was an American biochemist who in 1985 invented the polymerase chain reaction (PCR), a technique to amplify DNA sequences. He was awarded a Nobel Prize in Chemistry with **Michael Smith** in 1993.

Stanley Prusiner is an American neurologist who was awarded the Nobel Prize for his work on prions, "infectious proteins."

These innovative observations and inventions have contributed greatly to modern science and changed our understanding of infectious diseases. Based on these solid scientific discoveries and information, the knowledge of infectious diseases has presently been integrated into the concept of multiple causation of infectious diseases.

1.4 THE CONCEPT OF MULTIPLE CAUSATION OF DISEASES

Infectious diseases including parasitic diseases and their distributions do not depend on the causative organisms alone. They occur as a result of interactions between three factors, i.e., the **agent**, the **host**, and the **environment**. Thus, the interaction of nutritional, chemical, physical, or mechanical properties of the agent,

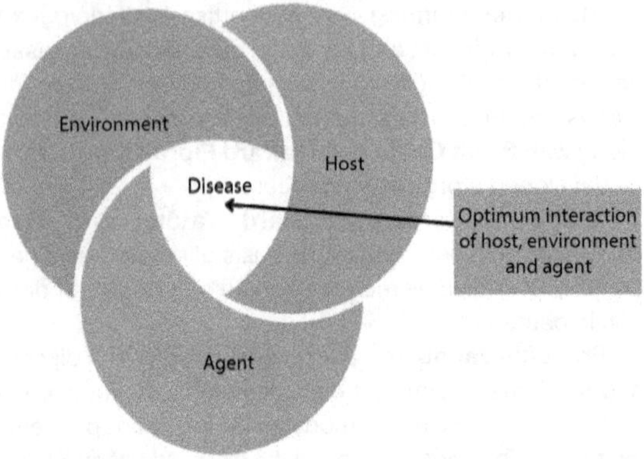

Figure 1.2 Factors that play a role in disease outbreak.

the age, sex, and race, and the genetic constitution of the host, as well as biological, social, economic, and physical changes in the environment, may play significant roles in disease occurrence.

This means that although all three of these units are necessary, none single-handedly is a sufficient cause of a disease. The interaction of these three factors largely determines one's state of health. The agent and the host are supported by the environment, which forms the fulcrum or lever.

The operation and interaction of these factors in equilibrium lead to health, whereas disease results when this equilibrium is disturbed by harmful alterations. Health and disease therefore are both determined by agent–host–environment interactions.

There is the need for the maintenance of a beneficial relationship between these three factors referred to as "**balanced pathogenicity.**" This tends to promote and prolong the health and survival of both the parasite and the host. Where parasite pathogenicity exceeds host defences, the health of the host is impaired, and parasite survival is promoted.

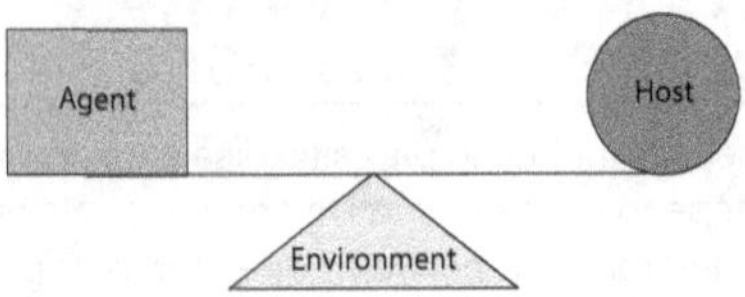

Figure 1.3 Agent–host–environment interactions.

TABLE 1.1 Agent–Host Interactions and Their Outcomes

Agent	*Interactions*	*Host*	*Outcome*
Parasite	*Parasite pathogenicity (More)* *Host defences (Less)*	Host	***Poor host survival***
Parasite	*Parasite pathogenicity (Less)* *Host defences (More)*	Host	***Poor parasite survival***
Parasite	*Parasite pathogenicity (Equal)* *Host defences (Equal)*	Host	***Enhanced survival of both***

1.5 HOST–PARASITE INTERACTIONS

1.5.1 ANIMAL ASSOCIATIONS

To understand medical parasitology, it is imperative to have a fair knowledge of animal associations. This refers to the situation where animals live interdependently of each other for food, shelter, or general survival. Technically, there are two types of animal associations, i.e., Homospecific/Homogenetic and Heterospecific/Heterogentic.

Homospecific *or homogenetic association*: Describes association between organisms of the same species or genotype, e.g., herds, colonies, flocks, etc.

Heterospecific *or heterogenetic association*: Describes association between different species or genotypes of animals. This is usually complex and has been described by several terms, e.g., symbiosis.

These animal associations can further be categorized as described in the following sections.

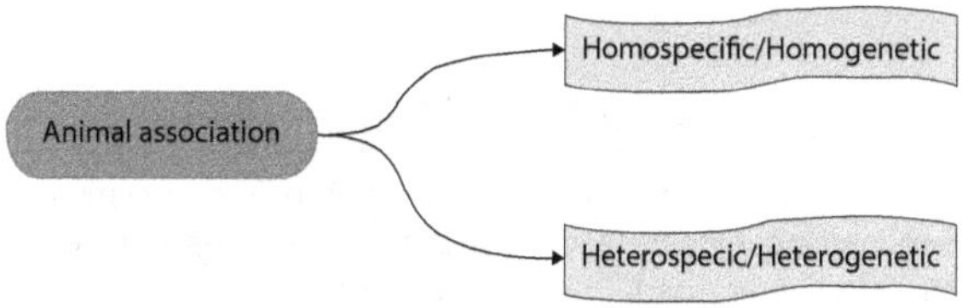

Figure 1.4 Animal associations.

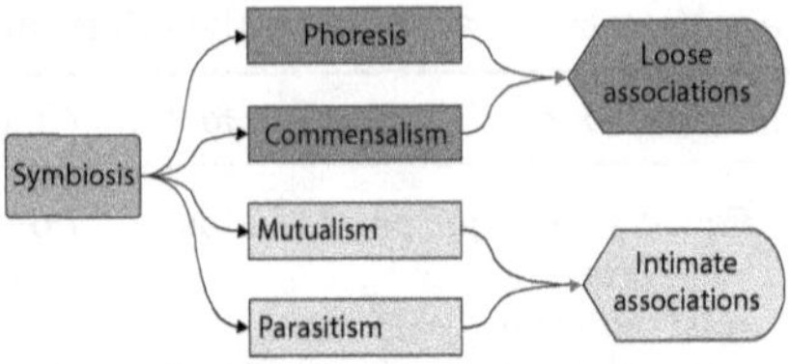

Figure 1.5 Types of symbiotic associations.

1.5.2 SYMBIOSIS (LIVING TOGETHER)

Any two organisms living in close association, commonly one living in/on the body of the other (A. de Bary 1879). This term has been used in diverse ways to describe animal associations. In simple terms, it means living together. This kind of relationship among animals involves various levels of intimacy. Depending on the level of intimacy, a symbiotic association could be referred to as Phoresis, Commensalism, Mutualism, or Parasitism. The symbionts (the organisms involved) usually differ in size.

1.6 TYPES OF SYMBIOTIC ASSOCIATIONS

1.6.1 PHORESIS AND COMMENSALISM

These represent loose associations; usually, there is no metabolic dependence; they are basically companionships.

1.6.1.1 Phoresis (Travelling Together)

Phoresis is an association in which two symbionts travel together. The host organism (usually the larger organism) merely provides shelter, support, or transport for the phoront (the smaller organism). There is no metabolic, physiological, or biochemical dependence, e.g., a) **sedentary protozoans**, algae, and fungi that attach to the bodies of aquatic arthropods, b) Fierasfer fish which thrive in the respiratory trees of holothurians/starfishes.

1.6.1.2 Commensalism (Eating at Table)

Commensalism is an association in which only one symbiont or commensal benefits by feeding on the food remains (leftover food) of the other (the host). The host is neither helped nor harmed. Usually, there is no metabolic or physiological dependence.

However, the host may provide shelter for the commensal. This association may be facultative or obligatory, e.g., *Entamoeba gingivalis/Trichomonas tenax* in the mouth of humans.

1.6.2 MUTUALISM AND PARASITISM

These are associations involving some amount of intimacy. Usually, the metabolism or physiology of one species is dependent on the other species.

1.6.2.1 Mutualism

Mutualism is an association in which both symbionts benefit. They are virtually inseparable and mutually dependent. This is usually obligatory, and there is metabolic or physiological dependence, e.g., a) the union between algae and fungi (Lichen) or b) flagellates and termites. The flagellates provide cellulase enzyme for the digestion of cellulose by the termites, and c) leeches and intestinal bacteria which aid in the digestion of blood.

1.6.2.2 Parasitism

Parasitism is an intimate and continuous relationship between two different organisms, usually of different species. This association involves both metabolic and physiological or biochemical dependence of the parasite on the host. The following observations are true concerning this kind of association.

- The parasite lives at the expense of the host.
- The host provides nutrients, shelter, and transport, etc., for the parasite.
- The parasites do not usually readily kill their host.
- Some parasites undergo part of their life cycles in the host.

The union between pathogenic agents and their host is a dynamic evolutionary process which represents various levels of symbiosis between different species of organisms.

The ***degree of dependence*** of a parasite on its host varies from one species to another, e.g., Malaria parasites (*Plasmodium falciparum, P. malariae, P. vivax,* and *P. ovale*) which are obligatory parasites cannot survive outside the host, whereas some helminth parasites which are free-living or facultative can live and

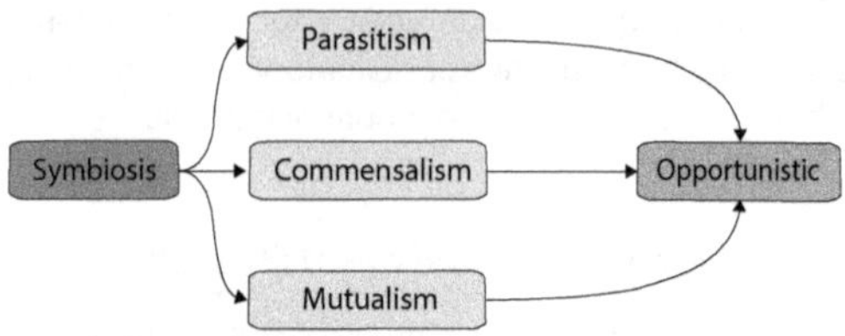

Figure 1.6 Levels of symbiotic associations between different organisms.

exist outside the host in the soil, e.g., hookworms (*Ancylostoma duodenale* and *Necator americanus*).

Parasitic infections ranging from innocuous to fatal conditions form a major part of tropical infectious diseases.

1.7 PARASITES AND PARASITISM

Parasites are organisms that live or reside in, on, or with(in) another organism, often referred to as the host, in order to obtain nutrients, grow, or multiply, usually in a state that directly or indirectly harms the host; in extreme cases, they may even cause death. There are three main classes of parasites that cause human infections:

1. *Protozoa*: Microscopic, one-celled organisms can be free-living or parasitic in nature. Examples include the malaria parasite and leishmaniasis parasites.
2. *Helminths*: Large, multicellular organisms that are generally visible to the naked eye in the adult stages. Examples include trematodes (flukes), cestodes (flatworms), and nematodes (roundworms).
3. *Ectoparasites*: Organisms that attach or burrow into the skin and remain there for a relatively longer period. Examples include ticks, fleas, lice, and mites.

1.7.1 PARASITES ARE EUKARYOTIC ORGANISMS

There are two primarily different types of cells, the eukaryotic cells and prokaryotic cells. Eukaryotic cells are far larger and more complex than prokaryotic cells. A prokaryotic cell has no true nucleus; its DNA lies free in a region in the cytoplasm called the

TABLE 1.2 Review of the Properties of Prokaryotic and Eukaryotic Cell

	Prokaryotic Cells	*Eukaryotic Cells*
Cellular organization	Simple	Complex
Cell size	Average diameter 0.5–10 μm	Average diameter 10–100 μm
Nucleus	No membrane	Membrane present with nucleolus
Chromosomes	Single circular chromosome	Multiple chromosomes
Extra chromosomal DNA	Often in the form of plasmids	Found in organelles
Nitrogen fixation	Possible for some	Impossible for all
Organelles in the cytosol	Few, without envelope	Many envelopes/membranes bound, e.g., mitochondria, nucleus, chloroplasts
Cytoplasmic membrane	Has a metabolic function. Contains enzymes needed of respiration, there is active secretion of enzymes, it is the centre for DNA synthesis and contains phospholipids	Has no metabolic function. It is a semi-permeable layer
Cell wall	Made up of a rigid peptidoglycan except in the case of Mycoplasma	No peptidoglycan but may contain polysaccharides, e.g., cellulose
Sterols	Absent except in Mycoplasma	Usually present
Ribosomes	70S in cytosol	80S in cytoplasmic reticulum
Form	Often unicellular	Unicellular/multicellular
Examples	Bacteria and viruses	Parasites

nucleoid, whereas a eukaryotic cell has a true membrane-bound nucleus, which contains the DNA.

Parasitism is a physiological association between two living organisms in which the host meets the nutritional and metabolic requirements of the parasitic organism.

1.8 TYPES OF PARASITES

i) *Ectoparasites*
Parasitic organisms that live on the outside (external) of their host, usually attached to the skin, hairs etc., e.g., fleas, lice, ticks, midges, etc. They are usually aerobic (utilize atmospheric O_2) and can live a completely non-parasitic existence.

ii) *Endoparasites*
Parasitic organisms that live within their hosts, in locations such as the gut, body cavity, blood, liver, lungs, tissues, etc. e.g., *Giardia lamblia*, *Entamoeba histolytica*, *Taenia solium*.
Some organisms fall into both groups, e.g., *Sarcoptes scabei*.

iii) *Facultative*
Parasitic organisms that do not depend on their host absolutely can live either a parasitic or non-parasitic existence. They become parasitic accidentally when ingested or when they gain access into wounds or other body orifices, e.g., *Naegleria fowleri* and *Strongyloides stercoralis*.

iv) *Obligate*
Parasitic organisms that depend absolutely on their hosts. Obligate parasites are obliged to live a parasitic existence and are incapable of surviving outside the host environment. These organisms, however, may have free-living stages outside the host, e.g., *Plasmodium* spp., *Entamoeba histolytica*, *Endolimax nana*.

v) *Opportunistic*
These organisms take advantage of changes in the host immune or physiological state to infect the host. They cause diseases in immunocompromised hosts, e.g., *Toxoplasma gondii*, *Cryptosporidium parvum*, *Isospora belli*, *Cyclospora cayetanensis*, *Microsporidia*, *Cryptococcus neoformans*, *Pneumocystis carinii* or *jiroveci*, and *Entamoeba* spp.

vi) *Accidental/incidental*
These are organisms that acquire an unusual/unnatural host and survive in that host. They usually do not survive in the wrong host, but when they do, they can be extremely

pathogenic, e.g., *Naegleria fowleri*, *Hymenolepis diminuta*, and *Toxocara canis* infection in humans.

vii) *Erratic*

Parasitic organisms that wander into unnatural sites. They normally invade body organs such as the brain, liver, and lungs of humans, e.g., *Entamoeba histolytica*.

viii) *Periodic or sporadic*

Organisms that parasitize their host intermittently to obtain some metabolic benefits.

Types of Parasites by Host Association and Life Cycle

i) *Temporary or intermittent*

These are parasitic organisms that feed on the host and leave. They are referred to as macropredators. They can prey on several hosts at a time, e.g., mosquitoes, bedbugs.

ii) *Monoxenous parasites*

These parasites require a single host to complete a life cycle.

iii) *Heteroxenous parasites*

These organisms need two or more different host species (a definitive host and intermediate hosts) to complete each life cycle.

iv) *Auto heteroxenous parasites*

These are parasites in which the definitive host of one generation becomes the intermediate host of the next generation.

v) *Spurious parasites*

These are free-living organisms which are accidentally introduced into a host and succeed in surviving therein for a time. Vinegar eels, *Turbatrix aceti*, introduced into the human vagina during douching, can maintain themselves there for a time. Parasites could also be referred to as one of the following in different contexts: pathogenic or non-pathogenic, invasive or non-invasive, virulent or avirulent, etc.

1.8.1 DEFINITION OF A HOST

The host is the larger of the two species in the symbiotic relationship and may be categorized as:

1. ***Definitive host/final host***: The host in which the developing parasite attains sexual maturity, e.g., mosquitoes in malaria infection.
2. ***Intermediate host***: The host that serves as a temporary environment for the growth and development of the parasite. *Bulinus truncatus* in *Schistosoma* infections. Arthropods

and other invertebrate organisms that serve as intermediate hosts are referred to as vectors.

3. ***Paratenic or transport/transfer host***: The host used as a temporary hideout until an appropriate definitive host is encountered, e.g., the larger freshwater fish that harbour the plerocercoid stage.

   In a paratenic host, the parasite remains alive and infective but does not undergo development; it usually forms an ecological bridge between an intermediate and definitive host. Some parasites show host specificity (preference for a particular host species).

4. ***Reservoir host***: The host that harbours parasites that could be transmitted to humans, e.g., wild cats that harbour *Trichinella spiralis*.

The main requirements for parasitism by infectious pathogens follow a common pattern. For example, the factors necessary for transmission and outcomes of host–parasite interactions are similar; secondly, not all infections lead to disease conditions. The advent of an infection may result in coexistence of the host and parasite, simple colonization of the host, or a small fraction of the infected individuals may develop overt (obvious/clinical) or covert (hidden/sub-clinical) conditions.

Similarly, the progression of infections to the eventual outcome of host–parasite interactions is similar and may depend to a

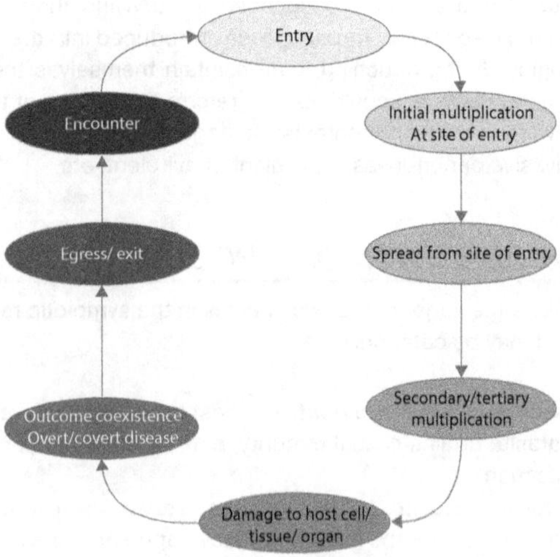

Figure 1.7 Events that occur from encounter of host to the eventual outcome of host–parasite–interactions.

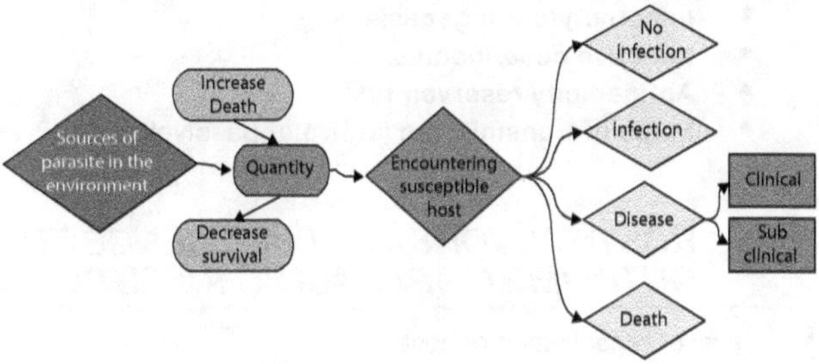

Figure 1.8 Progression of infections to the eventual outcome of host–parasite.

significant extent on the essential role of ligand–receptor interactions, pathogenesis, and immunological state of the host.

1.8.2 INFECTIONS

Each of the above events necessitates the breaching of host defence mechanisms, and different parasites elicit different host responses and may use different mechanisms to evade host immune responses.

1.9 HOST–PARASITE INTERRELATIONSHIPS

1.9.1 NATURE OF INFLUENCES OF PARASITES ON THE HOST

Medically important parasites exert varied influences on their host organisms. The nature of these influences may be simple or complex depending on an integration of parasite and host-related factors. These factors usually determine the outcome of an infection.

Parasite factors that influence the outcome of an infection:

- Species of parasite – this determines its level of organization/complexity:
  - **Physiology**
  - **Morphology**
- Capacity to cause disease in the host – this is based on the following characteristics:
  - **Virulence**
  - **Invasiveness**

- **Infectivity/pathogenesis**
- **Infective dose/inoculum**
- **Antigenicity reservoir host**
- **Mode of transmission (active or passive)**

1.9.2 HOST FACTORS THAT INFLUENCE THE OUTCOME OF PARASITIC INFECTIONS

- Level of organization of host
- Host response or reaction to infection/host genetic susceptibility
- Site of infection
- Incubation period
- Age/sex/nutritional status
- Behaviour/culture/socioeconomic status
- Level of education
- Underlying disease/condition (i.e., alcoholism, immunocompromised)
- Mobility (movement of host)
- Herd immunity, etc.

1.9.2.1 Examples of Influences of Parasites on Host

a. ***Mechanical disturbances*** (attachment/injuries/movements, *etc*.). This may lead to different degrees of cell/tissue/organ damage. Examples include:
    - Injuries resulting from the attachment of organs, e.g., the egg of trematodes, scolexes of cestodes, and buccal cavities of hookworms (the results of this could be very traumatic to the host).
    - Irritating movement of parasites within their hosts. Movement of cutaneous larval migrans.
    - Penetration of skin by larval stages of *Schistosoma* spp., hookworm, *Strongyloides stercoralis*.
    - Partial and complete obstruction of certain parts of the host, e.g., *Ascaris lumbricoides* blocking the alimentary canal, liver flukes blocking the bile duct, effects of filarial worms blocking the lymphatic system (elephantiasis), blocking of the pharynx and bronchial pipes by worms.
    - Exertion of pressure on tissues and organs such as the brain (leading to impairment of functions), e.g., worms aggregating and lodging in the kidneys, liver, and lungs, occupancy or aggregation of larval cestodes in tissues,

e.g., *Echinococcus granulosus* (Hydatid) cyst lodging and growing in the brain of humans.

- Bites of ectoparasites, etc., e.g., mosquitoes, bed bugs, ticks, mites. Mechanical action has a local effect, but injuries to a vital organ could lead to complications.

b. ***Interference with host metabolism***

This occurs due to the destruction and utilization of substances of the host required for normal development/metabolism, leading to the depletion of vital elements for the growth of the host. Common examples include the following:

- Use of host food (carbohydrates/glucose) and blood by malaria parasites.
- Secretion of anti-coagulants by vectors leading to loss of blood after feeding/bites.
- Use of host food components by parasites, e.g., fish tapeworm (*Diphyllobothrium latum*) competes with the host for vitamins A and B12. *D. latum* absorbs over 30 times the amount absorbed by other parasitic tapeworms, and its infection can lead to anaemia.
- Production of inhibitory substances for food uptake.
- Loss of blood by host as a result of increased worm burden, e.g., hookworm infection.
- Activities of hematophagous arthropods such as ticks, fleas, bugs, etc.
- Destruction of substances necessary for normal metabolism. This can have a significant effect on the gonads of the host and can lead to degeneration/complete atrophy.

c. ***Production of toxic substances***

This refers to the endo/exo toxins, poisons, and other secretions produced and introduced into the host by bacteria/viruses/parasites and arthropods. These substances elicit local or general immune reactions. Examples include:

- Toxic substances which give a general rather than local pathogenic response.
- Secretions of schistosomes that cause allergic/inflammatory reactions (cercarial dermatitis).
- Toxins that may be antigens that elicit host response.
- Toxins associated with changes in blood composition, such as a rise in eosinophilia (e.g., in hookworm infections) and the production of haemolytic substances by the parasites lead to a drop in RBC count.
- Toxins that are neurotoxic, e.g., substances produced by *Diphyllobothrium latum*, *Ascaris lumbricoides*, and *Trichuris trichiura*.

d. ***Promotion of other infections***

This involves the introduction of other organisms into the host body leading to secondary infections.

- Bacterial inflammation of the appendix due to the presence of *Trichuris trichiura* in the appendix.
- *Entamoeba histolytica/Balantidium coli* infections that give way for other bacterial (secondary) invasion as a result of the formation of ulcerations and tissue invasion.
- The migration of helminthic parasites that carry other organisms with them during migration, e.g., migration of *Ascaris lumbricoides* in the host body (larval migrans).

e. ***Sensitization – immune response of the host***

Movement of parasites within the host body may lower the immunity of the host.

1.10 ADAPTATIONS OF PARASITIC ORGANISMS

To thrive within or upon a host, parasites must overcome rigorous physiological barriers and environmental challenges. This section highlights the key structural, functional, and reproductive modifications that parasites have evolved to successfully navigate host defenses, secure attachment, and maximize their chances of transmission.

- ***Biological/physiological adaptation***
  Refers to the ability of parasites to withstand the action of host digestive juices and to alter their respiratory processes to extremely low oxygen tensions (e.g., intestinal worms).
- ***Atrophy or absence of organs***
  Loss or lack of specialized organs, i.e., digestive, defence/predatory, sensory, locomotory organs (e.g., flagella, cilia, pseudopodia) organs.
- ***Prolific reproductive function***
  Reproductive capacity of parasitic organisms is often very prolific to offset the unfavourable conditions encountered during their lifecycles in their host organisms/environment.
- ***Structural/anatomical modification***
  The modification of the cuticle of intestinal worms to carry out selective absorption and the evolution of suckers, hooks, and other organs of attachment are examples. Such organs are specifically useful in a parasitic existence.
- ***Modifications of the life cycle***
  To facilitate transmission from host to host, the life history is often profoundly modified and may become very complex.

Reproduction by immature forms in order to facilitate production of offspring in large numbers, the adoption of intermediate and paratenic hosts, and the correlation of the life history of the parasite with the habits and life history of these and of the definitive host may occur.

1.11 DEFINITIONS

Rickettsia *refers to a group of intracellular bacteria transmitted by arthropods that cause various febrile diseases in humans and animals.*

Prions *are proteinaceous infectious particles that cause fatal neurodegenerative diseases by inducing misfolding of normal brain proteins, leading to progressive brain damage and death.*

Viroids *are tiny, circular RNA molecules without protein coats that infect plants, causing serious diseases by disrupting normal cellular functions.*

Teleology *is the explanation of phenomena in terms of the purpose they serve, rather than solely focusing on the cause by which they arise, is also the belief that everything has a purpose.*

Fomites *are any inanimate object that, when contaminated with or exposed to infectious agents (such as pathogenic bacteria, viruses, or fungi), can transfer disease to a new host. These objects act as passive vectors, facilitating the transmission of pathogens.*

Miasmas *are an oppressive or unpleasant atmosphere that surrounds or emanates from something.*

Renaissance *refers to a period in European civilization that followed the Middle Ages. This period bridged the gap between the ancient world and the modern era by sparking curiosity, creativity, and intellectual exploration.*

Pasteurization *is a heat-treatment process used primarily in the food and beverage industry to destroy or deactivate pathogenic microorganisms and enzymes that cause spoilage and disease, thereby enhancing food safety and extending shelf life.*

Sterilization *is a process that completely destroys or eliminates all forms of microbial life, including bacteria, viruses, fungi, and spores, from an object or surface.*

Antiseptic *is a substance or chemical agent that slows, inhibits, or kills the growth of microorganisms – such as bacteria, viruses, or fungi – on the external surfaces of the body.*

Aetiology *is the study or science of the causes or origins of diseases or medical conditions. It involves investigating the factors that produce or predispose individuals to certain disorders or illnesses.*

Anaesthesia *is a medical intervention that induces a controlled, temporary loss of sensation or awareness to prevent pain and discomfort during surgical or medical procedures.*

Asymptomatic *refers to a medical condition or illness where a person carries the disease or infection but does not exhibit any symptoms throughout the course of the illness.*

Oncogene *is a gene that makes cells grow too much and too fast, which can lead to cancer. It comes from a normal gene called a proto-oncogene, but when changed, it acts like a stuck gas pedal causing uncontrolled cell division.*

Malignant tumours *are cancerous growths composed of cells that grow uncontrollably, invade nearby tissues, and have the ability to spread to distant parts of the body through the blood or lymphatic system.*

Balanced pathogenicity *refers to the delicate equilibrium between the harmful effects caused by pathogens and the host's ability to mount an effective immune response, determining the outcome of infection and disease progression in a dynamic interplay between pathogen virulence and host defences.*

PCR *is a foundational molecular biology technique used to amplify specific DNA sequences, producing millions to billions of copies from a small initial sample – aiding genetic research, medical diagnostics, forensic science, and even evolutionary biology.*

Sedentary protozoans *are a group of single-celled organisms within the protozoan phylum that exhibit limited or no motility and typically reside in a fixed location, often attached to substrates or surfaces, where they feed and reproduce, displaying adaptations suited to their stationary lifestyle.*

Algae *refer to a diverse group of photosynthetic organisms found in various aquatic environments.*

Fungi *refer to a kingdom of usually multicellular eukaryotic organisms that are heterotrophs, meaning they cannot produce their own food and must obtain nutrients from other organic sources.*

Degree of dependence of a parasite *refers to how much it relies on its host for survival and reproduction.*

"Free-living" or "facultative" *refer to protozoans that can exist and thrive independently in various environments without being obligatorily parasitic or symbiotic. These organisms* *have the capacity to move and feed on organic matter, bacteria, or other microorganisms in their surroundings, and they do not necessarily rely on a host for their survival. This lifestyle allows them to inhabit diverse habitats such as soil, freshwater, marine environments, and even moist terrestrial environments.*

"From innocuous to fatal" *refers to the range of impacts that parasitic infections can have on their hosts, varying from mild or asymptomatic to severe illness, organ damage, or even death, depending on factors such as the parasite species, host immunity, and the presence of underlying health conditions.*

Neurotoxic *refers to the ability of a substance or chemical to damage the brain or peripheral nervous system caused by exposure to natural or man-made toxic substances.*

Movement of parasites *has the tendency to interfere with the activity of white blood cells and thereby affect the general immunity of the host against both parasitic infections as well as other opportunistic infections.*

Haematophagous arthropods *are those that feed on blood. The term is derived from the Greek words "haima," meaning blood, and "phagos," meaning to eat.*

Atrophy *is a decrease in size of a body part, cell, organ, or other tissue due to factors like lack of use, ageing, or disease. The term implies that the atrophied part was of a size normal for the individual, considering age and circumstance, prior to the diminution.*

FURTHER READING

Bogtish, B. J., Carter, C. E., & Oeltmann, T. N. (2019). Chapter 1 – Symbiosis and parasitism. In B. J. Bogitsh, C. E. Carter, & T. N. Oeltmann (Eds.), *Human Parasitology* (5th ed., pp. 1–14). Academic Press. https://doi.org/10.1016/B978-0-12-813712-3.00001-1

Brooker, S., & Bundy, D. (2014). Soil-transmitted Helminths (Geohelminths). *Manson's Tropical Diseases*, 1515–1548. https://doi.org/10.1016/B978-0-7020-5101-2.00056-X.

Field, M. C. (2022). Molecular cellular parasitology: The decades and challenges ahead. *Frontiers in Parasitology*, 1, 963515.

Goater, T. M., Goater, C. P., & Esch, G. W. (2014). *Parasitism: The diversity and ecology of animal parasites.* Cambridge University Press.

Lane, N. (2015, 6 March). The unseen world: Reflections on Leeuwenhoek (1677) 'concerning little animal'. *Philosophical*

Transactions of the Royal Society B: Biological Sciences, 370, 1666.

Leventhal, R., & Cheadle, R. F. (2019). *Medical parasitology: A self-instructional text.* FA Davis.

Watson, J. M. (1965). *An introduction to parasitology.* Butterworth-Heinemann.

Winkelstein, W. (1995). A new perspective on John Snow's communicable disease theory. *American Journal of Epidemiology.* https://doi.org/10.1093/aje/142.Supplement_9.S3

2 Morphology and Classsification of Parasites

Being a genius is one percent inspiration and ninety-nine percent perspiration.

Thomas Edison

CHAPTER OUTLINE

In this chapter, you will be introduced to the fundamental characteristics of parasitic organisms, including their morphology, classification, and general characteristics. By understanding their structure and nature, you will gain insights into how to properly group the parasites and identify them.

- *Explore Major Groups of Parasites*: Dive into the two major groups of parasites, ectoparasites, and endoparasites, and understand their distinct habitats and interactions with hosts. Learn about protozoans and metazoans, and their significance in medical and clinical contexts.
- *Uncover Examples of Protozoan and Metazoan Parasites*: Explore a variety of protozoan and metazoan parasites, including their unique characteristics, habitats, and medical implications. From microscopic unicellular organisms to complex multicellular parasites, you will uncover the diverse array of parasites that inhabit different environments.
- *Investigate the Cell Structure of Parasites*: Delve into the cellular anatomy of parasites, including the nucleus, endoplasmic reticulum, Golgi apparatus, mitochondria, and other organelles. Understand how these structures contribute to the physiological functions and adaptations of parasitic organisms.
- *Examine the General Characteristics of Protozoan Parasites*: Learn about the remarkable diversity of protozoan parasites, their habitats, life cycles, and adaptations to various metabolic pathways. Explore their phylogenetic diversity, specialized surfaces/organelles, and unique modes of reproduction.
- *Understand General Characteristics of Metazoan Parasites*: Explore the world of metazoan parasites, including

DOI: 10.1201/9781003733935-2

nematodes, platyhelminthes, and arthropods. Investigate their anatomical features, reproductive strategies, and classification based on morphology and life cycle.

- *Dive into the Classification of Protozoan and Metazoan Parasites*: Examine the classification systems used to categorize protozoan and metazoan parasites, including morphological, biochemical, and molecular criteria. Understand the sub-phyla and phyla classifications, and the evolutionary relationships among parasitic organisms.
- *Learn about Medically Important Protozoan and Metazoan Parasites*: Gain insights into the classification and characteristics of medically important protozoan and metazoan parasites. Explore their transmission dynamics, host preferences, and clinical manifestations in human populations

2.1 GENERAL STRUCTURE AND NATURE OF PARASITES

Parasitic infections are common everywhere but are more common in the tropical and subtropical areas of the world, where they are associated with significant rates of morbidity and mortality. It is important to acquire fundamental knowledge about their structure/nature, biology, genetics, metabolism, and behaviour to develop cogent approaches to control their infections and to develop effective drugs and vaccines.

2.1.1 MAJOR GROUPS OF PARASITES

There are two major groups of parasites: **Ectoparasites** and **endoparasites**. Ectoparasites are those that live outside the host, whereas endoparasites are those that live within the host. Endoparasites of medical/clinical importance can further be divided into two groups: Protozoans (unicellular organisms) and metazoans (multicellular organisms).

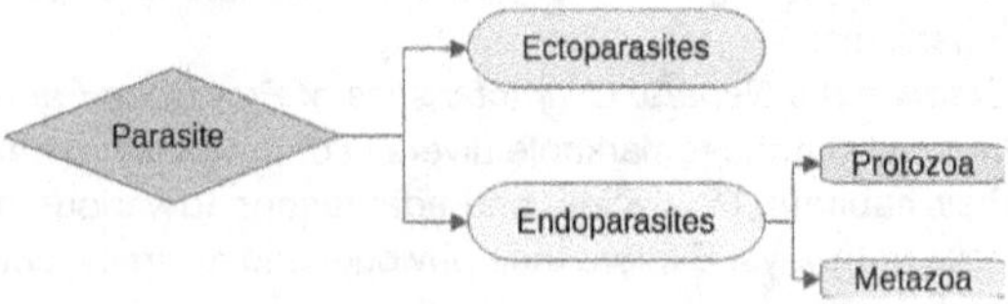

Figure 2.1 Examples of protozoan parasites.

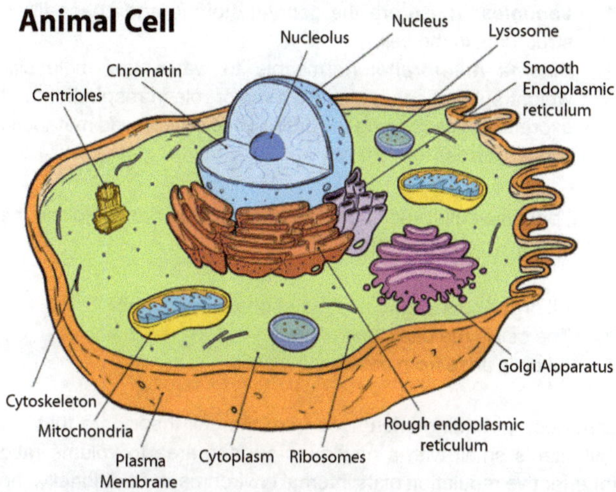

Figure 2.2 Structure of an animal cell.

2.1.1.1 BASIC MORPHOLOGY OF PARASITES

Parasites have a complex cellular organization. They are either unicellular or multicellular and function together. The cell of a parasite is similar to the animal cell and has the basic structure of an animal cell.

Like all animal cells, cells of parasites have a plasma membrane surrounded by cytoplasm and possess membrane-bound organelles, including the following:

- ***Nucleus with its nucleolus and chromosomes***: This contains the genetic material (DNA and chromosomes) needed for controlling cellular activities via genes.
- ***Nucleolus***: This region is located within the nucleus and is the site for ribosome synthesis.
- ***Rough endoplasmic reticulum (with ribosomes)***: This organelle is involved in protein synthesis.
- ***Smooth endoplasmic reticulum (without ribosomes)***: This organelle is involved primarily in lipid synthesis.
- ***Golgi apparatus***: This is the packaging centre for molecules and carbohydrate synthesis.
- ***Lysosomes***: This organelle contains hydrolytic enzymes for intracellular digestion.
- ***Mitochondria***: This is the site for ATP production and the energy-producing centre in the cell.

- ***Vacuoles***: These are the general storage and space-filling structures in the cell.
- ***Plasma membrane***: Permeable to water, low molecular weight substances and plays a major role in respiration and excretion by facilitating the diffusion of oxygen and metabolic wastes across its surface.

Thus, parasite cells, such as those of other eukaryotes, follow the cell theory, which infers that:

- All organisms are composed of one or more cells.
- The cell is the basic unit of life.
- All cells arise from pre-existing cells

Other compounding inferences from the cell theory are that the cell size is small with a maximum surface area to volume ratio for effective regulation of its internal environment. Additionally, the cell (plasma) membrane is composed of a fluid-like phospholipid bilayer, proteins, cholesterol, and glycoproteins, and the cell has a cytoplasm, which is the material outside the nucleus.

The cytoplasm contains organelles, which are membrane-bound sub-units of the cell with specialized functions. It is also the site for metabolic activities and is filled with the cytosol, a solution with dissolved substances, e.g., glucose, CO_2, and O_2.

Finally, there is the presence of a cytoskeleton, a supportive and metabolic structure composed of microtubules, microfilaments, and intermediate filaments.

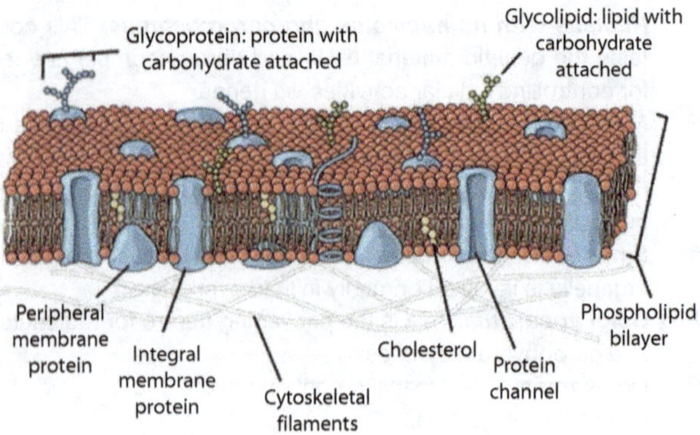

Figure 2.3 Section of the cell membrane.

2.2 CLASSIFICATION OF PROTOZOAN PARASITES

The classification of protozoa is under constant review because of recent important research findings, and different systems have been employed in the classification of these organisms. Different authors and scientists originally classified protozoan parasites on the basis of the following:

- Morphological characteristics determined through microscopy using, e.g., light, scanning, electron microscopes.
- Biochemical methods, e.g., isoenzyme analysis for stain identifications.
- Molecular probes, e.g., PCR, etc.

The sub-kingdom Protozoa has been divided into four phyla – Sarcodina, Mastigophora, Ciliophora, and Apicomplexa. Members of the first three phyla possess either pseudopodia, flagella, or cilia as locomotory organelles at some point in their life cycle. Members of the Apicomplexa group usually have no locomotory organelles in their definitive stage. The nuclei in the first three phyla are vesicular and vary in number between one and many. Members of the Ciliophora group usually have two compact nuclei (micro- and macronuclei).

Cilia and flagella are similar in structure; they are composed of microtubules (9+2), which form an axoneme surrounded by plasma membrane and anchored to the cell by the kinetosome. Flagella are usually in pairs, whereas cilia are generally numerous. Pseudopodia are cytoplasmic protrusions that aid in movement. Movement involves the use of actin, myosin, and ATP and involves changes in the fluid nature of the cytoplasm either from a solid (plasmagel – ectoplasm) state or a more fluid (plasmasol – endoplasm) state.

2.2.1 GENERAL CHARACTERISTICS OF PROTOZOAN PARASITES

Protozoans are found in almost every possible habitat, and all humans have protozoa living in/on their body at one time or another or are infected with a protozoan parasite throughout their lifetime. Diseases caused by protozoan parasites range from unapparent or mild to life-threatening presentations, particularly in immunosuppressed patients.

Protozoans are generally microscopic in size, but some, e.g., trophozoites of *Balantidium coli*, could be macroscopic and can

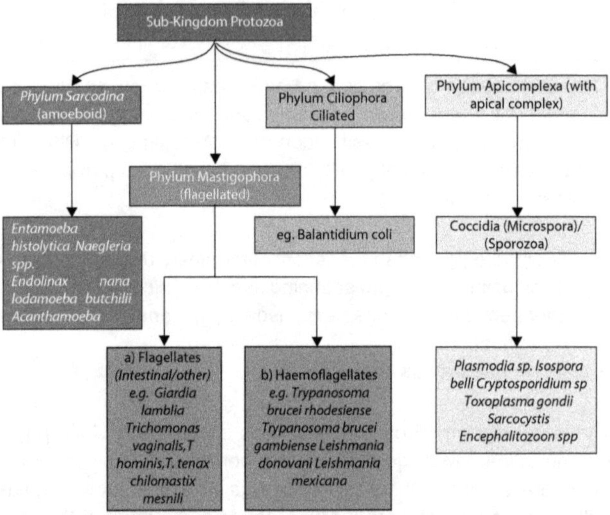

Figure 2.4 Classification of medically important protozoan parasites.

be seen with the naked eye. These organisms, like other higher animals, are equipped with structures or organelles that are specialized for essential functions needed for the maintenance of life. Protozoan parasites are unique for reasons including the following:

- They are single-celled, i.e., unicellular (one-celled) or sometimes referred to as acellular (cell-less) eukaryotes.
- They have a range of sizes, usually less than 50 µm. The smallest (mainly intracellular forms) are between 1 and 10 µm.
- They have different morphological forms and could be spherical, oval, bizarre, or shapeless depending on the class/group.
- They could be visible (macroscopic) or may require magnification (microscopic)
- They have membrane-bound nuclei.
- Other than ciliates (e.g., *Balantidium coli*), all protozoa have vesicular nuclei (bladder-like, bubble-like, pouch, usually fluid-filled) with scattered chromatin material that gives a diffuse appearance to the nuclei.
- They may have vesicular nuclei that contain a central body called the endosome or karyosome. The endosome lacks DNA in parasitic amoeba and trypanosomes.
- Those that belong to the Apicomplexa group have vesicular nuclei containing one or more nucleoli-containing DNA.

- Those belonging to the ciliate group have both micro and macro (somatic and germinal) nuclei.
- They have projecting locomotory structures such as pseudopodia, cilia, and flagella.
- They maintain their distinctive shapes via their rigid outer surface layer called the pellicle.
- They have cytoplasm differentiated into ectoplasm (outer transparent layer) and endoplasm (inner layer – sometimes granular, containing organelles).
- Those in the ciliate group, e.g., *Balantidium coli*, have cytostomes (cell mouths) for ingesting fluids or solid particles
- They may have contractile vacuoles for osmoregulation, e.g., *Naegleria fowleri*.
- They may be bilateral or radial in symmetry.
- They generally have organelles, a compact nucleus which contains genetic information, vesicles, Golgi apparatus, mitochondria, lysosomes, and food vacuoles, which are essential for life, reproduction, and also for physiological purposes.
- Trichomonads and trypanosomes have undulating membranes.
- Trypanosomes and *Leishmania* have kinetoplasts from which arise the flagella.
- They may undergo either sexual or asexual reproduction.
- They may have cytostomes (cell mouths) which are used for the ingestion of food, and undigested food may be expelled through a cytoproct (cell anus).
- They have endoskeletons that are formed from microtubular cytoskeletons of the cytoplasm.
- They have food vacuoles (phagosomes) containing ingested food substances enveloped by the plasma membrane; these food substances are obtained by phagocytosis.

2.2.2 CHARACTERISTICS OF MEMBERS OF THE SUB-PHYLUM SARCODINA

- They are shapeless organisms.
- They move by means of pseudopodia (cytoplasmic protrusions).
- Their body is divided into ectoplasm (clear) and endoplasm (granular).
- They reproduce by simple binary fission.
- They feed on particulate food, leading to the formation of food vacuoles.
- Their food is digested into glycogen.
- The infective stage is the cyst.

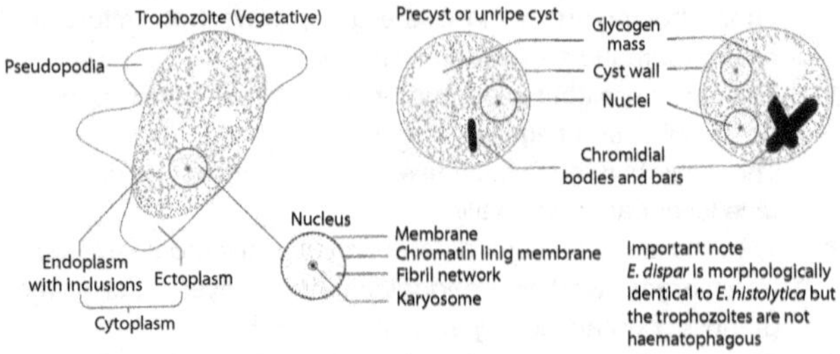

Figure 2.5 Diagram of *E. histolytica*.

- Chromatid bodies are bead-like karyosomes that are usually small and compact presence of RBCs (of diagnostic value).

2.2.3 CHARACTERISTICS OF MEMBERS OF THE SUB-PHYLUM MASTIGOPHORA

- They are elongated or torpedo-shaped.
- They move by means of flagella.
- Their reproduction is by binary fission.
- They inhabit the digestive tract, circulatory system, and tissues of their hosts.
- They require a liquid medium and are adapted to living in the blood, lymph, and cerebrospinal fluid.
- Forms such as *Leishmania* spp. have additional characteristics, i.e., kinetoplast.
- In the hemoflagellate group, common examples have a single flagellum and are transmitted by biting flies.
- The transmission of intestinal forms occurs via the ingestion of viable cysts.
- Transmission of *Trichomonas vaginalis*, however, is by sexual contact.

Undulating membrane bordered by a flagellum, 4–5 anterior flagella for movement Axostyle, which extends beyond the body.

2.2.4 CHARACTERISTICS OF MEMBERS OF THE SUB-PHYLUM CILIOPHORA

- Move by means of cilia.
- Have two dissimilar nuclei (micro and macro).
- Reproduce by binary fission.
- Have contractile and food vacuoles.

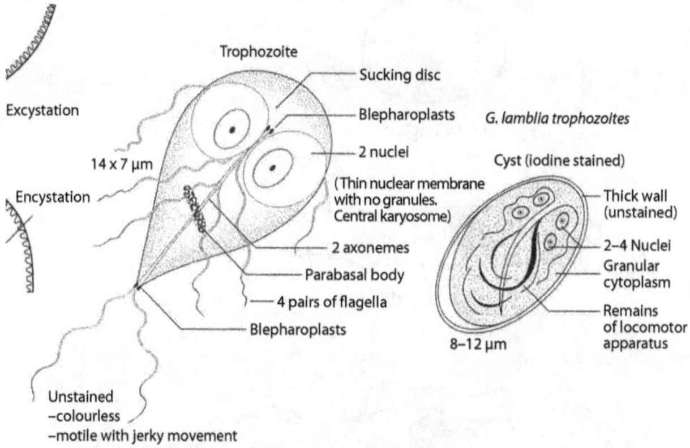

Figure 2.6 Diagram of the trophozoite and cyst of *Giardia lamblia*.

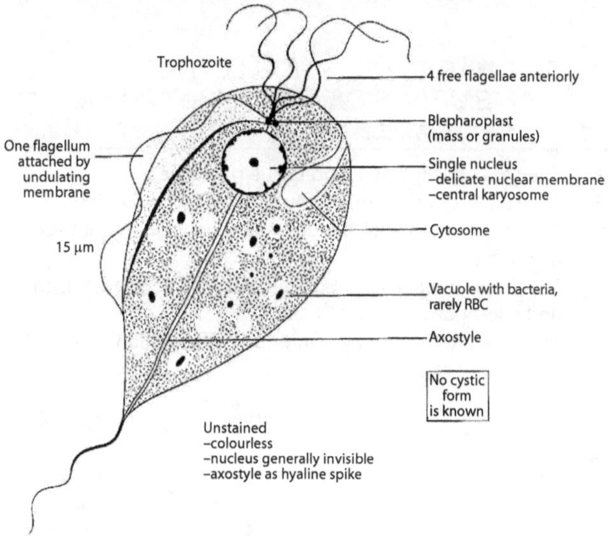

Figure 2.7 Diagram of *Trichomonas* spp.

- The infective stage is the cyst.
- Have cytostomes (cell mouth), cytopharynx, and cytophage.

Presence of cilia. Presence of micro/macro nuclei. Presence of cytostome/cytopharynx.

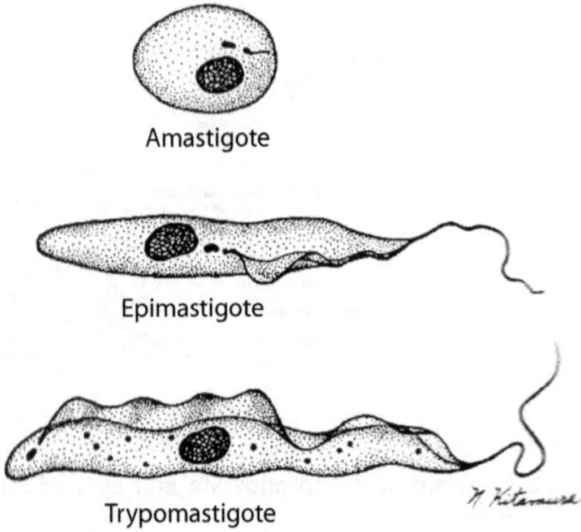

Figure 2.8 Morphological forms of trypanosomes.

2.2.5 CHARACTERISTICS OF THE MEMBERS OF THE SUB-PHYLUM APICOMPLEXA

- They are usually organ and tissue parasites.
- They have an apical complex consisting of polar rings.
- They have rhoptries, micronemes, conoids, and sub-pellicular tubules.
- Their reproduction is by both asexual and sexual (schizogony and sporogony).
- They are transmitted by arthropods or ingestion of oocysts.

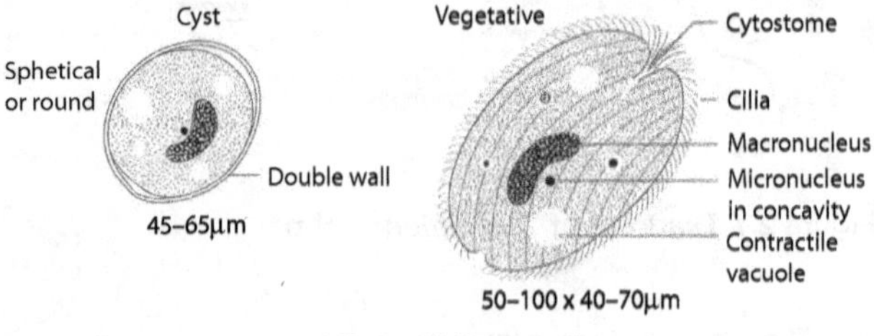

Figure 2.9 Diagram of *Balantidium coli*.

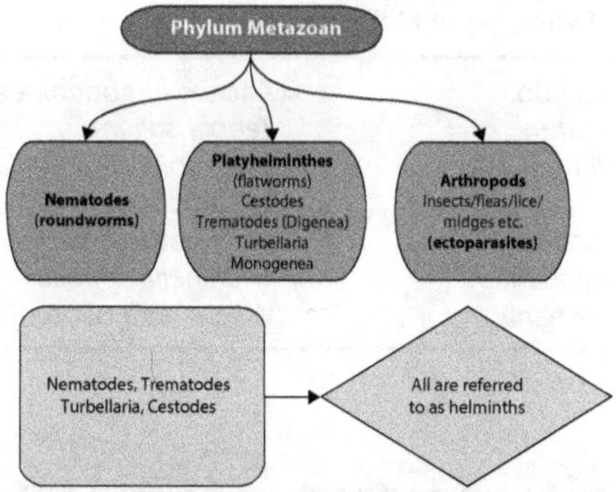

Figure 2.10 Classification of metazoans.

2.3 CLASSIFICATION OF METAZOAN PARASITES

Metazoan parasites are normally referred to as helminthes (Greek word meaning worm-like). These include nematodes (roundworms), the platyhelminthes (flatworms), and arthropods of medical importance.

The platyhelminthes and nematodes that infect humans have similar anatomic features that reflect common physiological requirements and functions, and the clinically relevant groups are separated according to their external shape and the host/organ of preference.

2.3.1 GENERAL CHARACTERISTICS OF METAZOAN PARASITES

- They are hermaphroditic and bisexual species.
- They are classified based on the external and internal morphological features of the egg (ova), larvae, and adults.
- They are generally invertebrates with round, flat, or elongated bodies.
- They develop through egg, larval (juvenile), and adult stages, known to have an outer covering (the tegument or cuticle), such as the flukes and tapeworms that have external features that include acetabula (suckers) or bothria (false suckers, also referred to as grooves),

2.3.2 GENERAL CHARACTERISTICS OF THE PHYLUM PLATYHELMINTHES

- They are dorsoventrally compressed.
- They are bilaterally symmetrical.

TABLE 2.1 Examples of Metazoan Parasites

Schistosoma spp.	*Ascaris lumbricoides*
Taenia saginata	*Taenia solium*
Diphyllobothrium spp.	*Enterobius vermicularis*
Loa loa	*Onchocerca volvulus*
Trichuris trichiura	*Ancylostoma duodenale*
Necator americanus	*Trichinella spiralis*
Hymenolepis nana	*Wuchereria bancrofti*

- They have a tegument which is **syncytial** (a multi-nucleated mass of protoplasm which is not subdivided into individual cellular components).
- They depend on diffusion for the removal of oxygen, nutrients and metabolic wastes. The diffusion occurs through the coelomic fluid.
- Their cephalic or anterior end is modified for attachment.
- They have an incomplete digestive tract/system with only one opening but several branches.
- Some members have no digestive tract.
- They have an excretory system that is bilaterally symmetrical and made up of tubules that terminate in flame cells (protonephridia), which are for osmoregulation.
- They lack a circulatory system.
- They have a nervous system consisting of **oesophageal commissures**.
- They have a reproductive system which is highly elaborated and complicated.
- Most are hermaphroditic – monoecious.
- In some cases, the sexes are separate and dioecious.
- Some exhibit asexual reproduction during their life cycle.
- Their life cycle is usually short, and development involves a single obligatory host; in some cases, however, there may be two hosts.
- They are transmitted through contaminated water, faeces or urine, containing infection agents – also auto-infection occurs, but may be rare.
- They are successful parasites because they could have self-fertilization although cross-fertilization is the general rule.
- Their worn-out sex organs are replaced constantly.
- They produce large numbers of eggs and have multiplication of larval stages, i.e., polyembryology – common among the flukes.

- They principally inhabit – lumen of the intestine, the respiratory system, blood vessels, visceral, and some may be found in the skin.
- Platyhelminthic forms are exclusively parasitic and include trematodes (flukes), cestodes (tapeworms), and free-living turbellarians.
- They are **triploblastic acoelomates**, i.e., they have three different tissue layers – the mesoderm, the ectoderm, and an endoderm. The mesoderm lies between the ectoderm and the endoderm. Their mesoderm is solid, muscular, and lacks a coelom (cavity); hence they are referred to as acoelomates.
- They are bilaterally symmetrical; as such, they are highly specialized organisms with both anterior and posterior ends, lateral/marginal sides, and also ventral and dorsal sides. The mouths are ventrally positioned.
- They are known to possess well-specialized organ systems such as the excretory, nervous, and reproductive systems. The reproductive system has structures such as the testes, ovaries, vas deferens, seminal vesicles, oviduct, and vitelline glands.

2.3.3 CHARACTERISTICS OF CLASS TREMATODA

- They are exclusively parasitic.
- Their larvae (miracidium) hatch from operculated/nonoperculated eggs and are usually ciliated. Adult stages have a tegument without cilia.
- They are leaf-like in shape.
- They range in length from a few mm to 7 or 8 cm.
- They have suckers for attachment (oral and ventral acetabula).

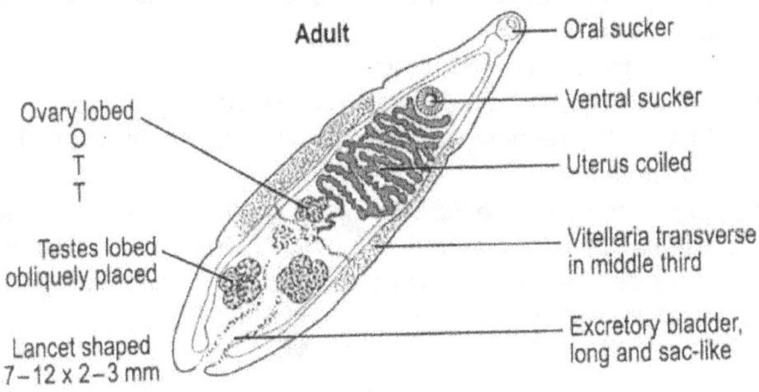

Figure 2.11 A typical drawing of an adult trematode.

- They lack a body cavity, and organs are embedded in connective (parenchyma) tissues.
- They have a digestive canal but lack an anus.

2.3.4 CHARACTERISTICS OF THE SUB-CLASS DIGENEA

- Digenea are mostly endoparasitic.
- They are mostly inhabitants of the vertebrate alimentary canal or may be associated with organs like the liver, bile duct, gall bladder, lungs, pancreatic duct, ureter, and bladder (organs with cavities and rich in semi-solid food materials, e.g., blood, mucus, and bile).
- They have organs of attachment (oral or circumoral) acetabulum.
- Their excretory pore is located at the posterior end of the body.
- They have a complicated developmental cycle with alternation of three or four generations – there is alternation of hosts during this time.
- Examples include *Fasciola hepatica*, *F. gigantica*, *Clonorchis*, *Opisthorchis*, *Fascioloides magna*, and *Dicrocoelium dendriticum*.

2.3.5 CHARACTERISTICS OF SCHISTOSOMES

- Sexes are separate.
- They are dimorphic.
- They have in portal blood system of vertebrates.
- Schistosomes, unlike other trematodes, have no pharynx.
- Schistosome eggs, unlike those of other trematodes, are not operculated.
- Larval forms have no pharynx.
- Schistosomes lack the metacercaria stage.
- They enter the host (definitive or final) directly through skin penetration.
- In humans, we have *Schistosoma mansoni* and *Schistosoma haematobium*, which are common in Ghana, *Schistosoma japonicum* – Asia, *Schistosoma mekongi* – Thailand, and *Schistosoma intercalatum* – Central Africa

2.3.6 CHARACTERISTICS OF PARAGONIMUS (LUNG FLUKE)

- They are small or medium-sized.
- They can be found in biliary/pancreatic passages; they can also be found in the lungs of vertebrates.
- Their eggs are small/medium-sized but have an operculum.
- Miracidium is well developed when eggs are laid.
- Cercariae produced from molluscs encyst into metacercaria in crustaceans, on vegetation, or in molluscs.

2.3.7 CHARACTERISTICS OF CLASS CESTODA (TAPEWORMS)

- Adults consist of a few or chains of many reproductive units (proglottids).
- They are flattened and elongated.
- They vary in length from 3 mm to 10 m.
- They may have three to several thousand segments.
- Their bodies are made up of the scolex (head region), neck/ strobila.

Scolex:

- It is usually pear-shaped (pyriform) or globular.
- It forms the anterior or cephalic end.
- It contains the cephalic ganglion or "brain" of the nervous system.
- It also bears the holdfast. It is used for attachment to the intestinal walls of the host.
- Grooved types are elongated. The sucker type is cup-like with four cutting discs. There may be an anterior protuberance (rostellum).
- The rostellum is retractile and cone-like – it may possess a crown of powerful hooks or spines.

Neck region of growth:

- It is situated behind the Scolex.
- It is unsegmented and a poorly differentiated area.
- It is narrower than the rest of the body.
- The posterior portion is the region of growth where new proglottids are produced and added to the body.

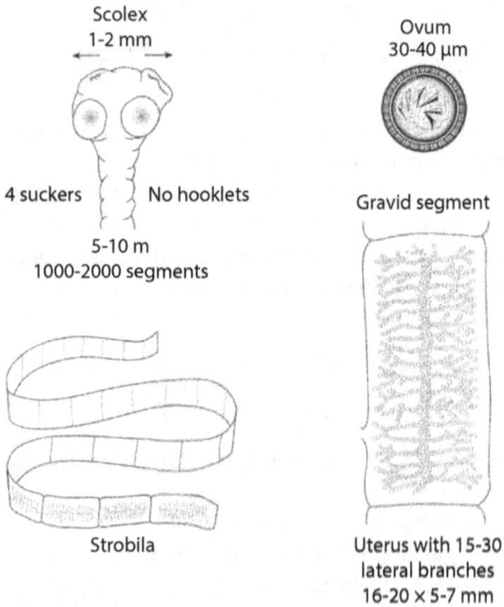

Figure 2.12 Diagram showing the various structures of cestodes.

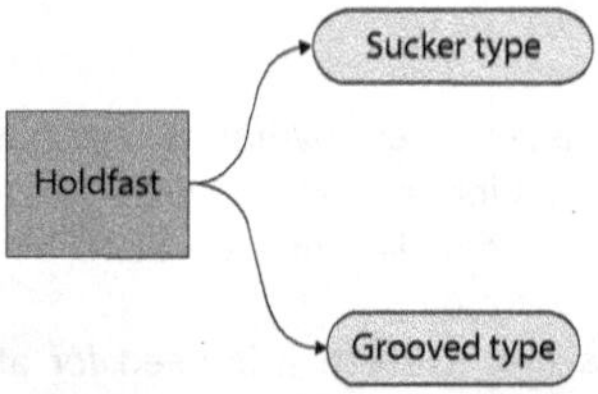

Figure 2.13 Illustration showing two attachment structures: A holdfast (left) and a grooved type sucker (right).

Strobila:

- This constitutes the rest of the body.
- It is made up of proglottids.
- The length of strobila varies in different cestodes – Usually 3–10 mm.
- The number may vary from 3,000 to 4,000.
- They are monoecious (each proglottid contains both male/ female sex organs).
- Internal organs help in the identification of the proglottid.

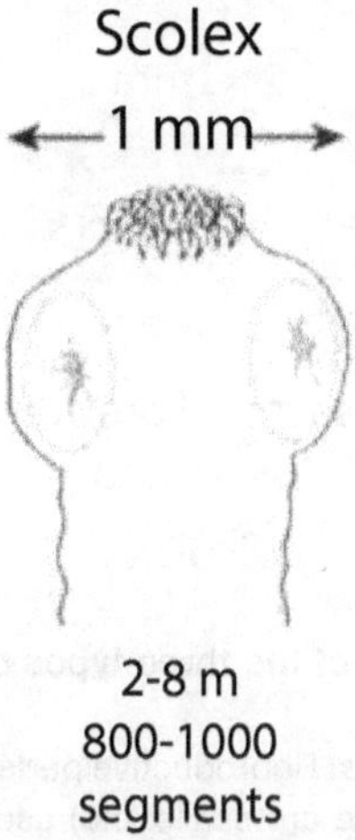

Figure 2.14 Diagram of the three types of scolices.

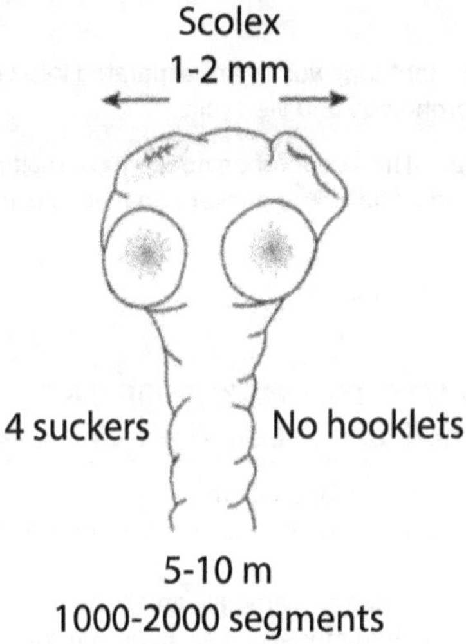

Figure 2.15 Diagram of the three types of scolices.

a) ***Immature***: Is distal to the neck in position, sex organs are not fully developed.
b) ***Mature***: Forms with full complements of the reproductive organs – sexually mature (they are ripe).

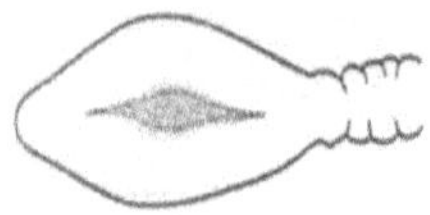

Figure 2.16 Diagram of the three types of scolices.

c) ***Gravid proglottids***: Reproductive parts are made up of egg-filled uterus. These are senile (old) usually the most posterior proglottid is the one that matures (gravid) first and these are shed into the intestine. This kind of shedding is called ecdysis.

Medically important tapeworms are separated into two groups on account of morphology and life cycle.

Cycophyllidean: This group of cestodes have multiple proglottid "segments." and all have four suckers on their scolices (heads).

Pseudophyllidean: This group has multiple segments and two bothria or sucking grooves.

2.3.8 CHARACTERISTICS OF THE PSEUDOPHYLLIDEAN GROUP

- Their eggs have an operculum.
- They have a more complex life cycle involving more than one host.
- They are parasites of mammals and birds.
- They have a characteristic vitelline pore through which eggs are released.
- The reproductive organs are concentrated in the middle of the proglottid, e.g., fish tapeworm, *Diphyllobothrium latum* (*Dibothriocephalus latus*), and *Spirometra* spp.
- Their lengths vary from 3 mm to 10 m.
- Scolex bears two sucking grooves (i.e., dorsal and ventral bothria).

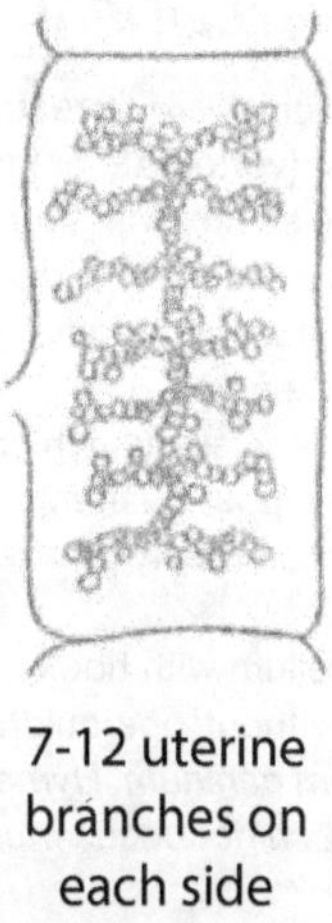

Figure 2.17 Illustration showing 7–12 uterine branches on each side of the structure.

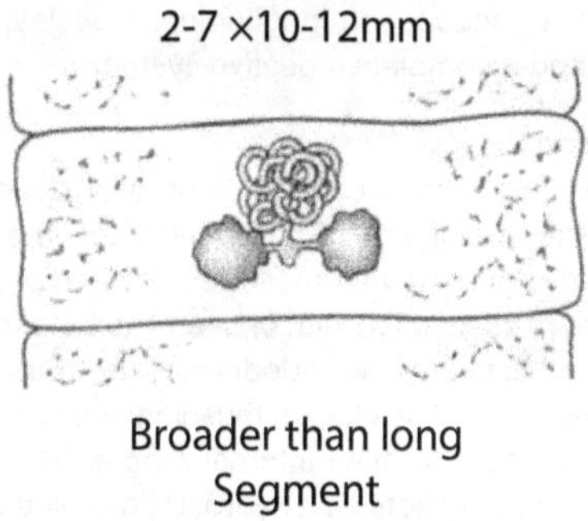

Figure 2.18 Illustration showing a segment that is broader than long, measuring 2–7 mm × 2–12 mm.

- Genital apertures are ventrally placed but could be lateral or dorsal.
- Testes and vitellaria are scattered and tend to encircle the other organs.
- The life cycle includes procercoid and plerocercoid stages.
- The first intermediate host is typically an aquatic invertebrate, while the second intermediate host is either a fish or a reptile.
- Their proglottids are usually longer than wide.

2.3.9 CHARACTERISTICS OF THE CYCLOPHYLLIDEAN GROUP

- They have an exclusively terrestrial life cycle with a single intermediate host (vertebrate or invertebrate).
- The head bears a scolex with four suckers.
- Their proglottids are usually wider than they are long.
- Their genital aperture is marginally placed.
- They lack a uterine pore.
- They have a single vitellaria, which is compact and lies posterior to the ovary (post-ovarian).
- Their larvae are commonly referred to as bladder worms or cysticercoid.
- They have a rostellum with hooks.
- Their eggs are without operculum, e.g., *Taenia saginata*, *T. solium*, *Dipylidium caninum*, *Hymenolepis nana*, *H. diminuta*, *Multiceps* spp., *Echinococcus multilocularis*, *E. granulosus*.

2.4 GENERAL CHARACTERISTICS OF PHYLUM NEMATODA

Some of the defining characteristics of nematodes include the possession of a pseudocoel, longitudinal muscles, a non-living outer cuticle, and a complete digestive system.

a) ***Pseudocoel***:
This is not a true body cavity. It is not well defined, as in the case of the coelomates. The pseudocoel is a body cavity that is not fully lined with mesoderm. The mesoderm in this case is more associated with or seems to be derived from the ectoderm than from the endoderm. Due to these structural alterations, nematodes lack a muscular lining of the gut, and mesenteries support their internal organs. The fluid that fills this pseudo cavity acts as a hydrostatic skeleton.

b) ***Longitudinal muscles***:
Roundworms, unlike other invertebrates, have only longitudinal muscles. The alterations and contractions of these muscles affect the shape of the organisms and explain the wavelike movement of their bodies. With a fluid-filled pseudocoel acting as a hydrostatic skeleton, the contraction of the longitudinal muscles alters the shape of the organisms and leads to observed whip-like and wavelike undulations seen spanning the entire length of the organism.

c) ***Non-living outer cuticle***:
Roundworms have a collagenous non-living outer covering produced by the epidermis called the cuticle. The cuticle

covers the external surface and also lines the buccal cavity of the oesophagus, as well as other body apertures. It is resistant to the digestive enzymes of the host and impervious to most substances except water and a few minute ions in aqueous solution. The cuticle functions as part of the hydrostatic skeleton and is able to resist high internal pressures posed by the pseudocoelomic fluid. The cuticle is made up of collagen and has three layers that form a lattice or mesh of fibres: The cortical layer, the median matrix layer, and the basal layer.

I. ***The cortical layer (epicuticle)***:
   This layer is antigenic. The glycocalyx may contain antibody–antigen complexes. It is composed of lipids, proteins and traces of carbohydrates. There is a metabolically active internal cortical layer that contains enzymes and RNA.
II. ***The median matrix layer***:
   This layer is made up of proteins resembling collagens. It may be filled with fluids and may also have structures such as rods, filaments and plates that allow the cuticle to be flexible longitudinally or strong radially.
III. ***The basal layer***:
   This layer contains fibres and has the same chemical composition as collagen.

d) ***Complete digestive system***:
   Nematodes have a complete digestive tract with an anterior opening (mouth) and a posterior opening (anus). This arrangement brings about a form of specialization (including changes in acidity and alkalinity) along the various regions of the digestive tract that allows the organism to process its food in a linear progressive sequence. Nematodes are generally referred to as roundworms. As a group, they are usually uniform in structure but differ in size and habitat preference. For example, hookworms *(Ancylostoma duodenale*, *Necator americanus)*, *Strongyloides stercoralis*, and *Ascaris lumbricoides* prefer to be in the ileum, *Trichuris trichiura* (whipworm) prefers to be in the colon, while *Enterobius vermicularis* (pinworm, seat worms) prefers to be in the caecum.

2.4.1 CHARACTERISTICS OF NEMATODES

Nematodes are:

- Pseudocoelomates.
- They have bodies filled with fluid in which body organs float.
- The fluid in their bodies functions as a hydrostatic skeleton.

- They are elongated and cylindrical, and taper at the posterior and anterior ends.
- They are unsegmented and lack external appendages.
- They are bilaterally symmetrical.
- They are covered with a tough protective covering or cuticle.
- Their sexes are separate – dioecious – they are also dimorphic, and the females are larger than the males.
- They possess a complete alimentary canal – fully functional.
- They have a tube, usually consisting of an aperture, a mouth cavity (buccal cavity).
- There is an oesophagus.
- Their intestine is flat, tube-like.
- Their anus is sub-terminal.
- When the mouth cavity is present, it may have teeth or cutting plates that have not been developed for sucking.
- The outer layer of the body forms a multi-layered proteinaceous cuticle containing collagen (protein) fibres, which allow contraction/extension of the body.
- They have no circulatory system – circulatory system function is done by fluid in the body, proteins, salts, glucose, vitamins, haemoglobin, etc.
- Their reproductive system is well developed.

The male system is well developed with spicules, vesicles, ejaculatory structures, vas deferens, testes, etc. It has one or two bristle-like, sclerotinized structures in the outer genital chamber of males, which are introduced into the vulva of females during copulation.

In some species – e.g., hookworm – males have a ring-like structure or appendage (bursae) which aids in copulation.

Females have a well-developed vulva, vagina, ovary, uterus, oviducts, etc.

- Daily egg output per female ranges from 200 to 250,000.
- They have a nervous system – dorsal/ventral nerves.
- They have an excretory system made up of two canals.
- They have muscles – feeding/contractile portions.
- Attachment is by attaching the oral part of the body to the host mucosa. Use oral bursae containing teeth. In Trichuris, the anterior end is thin and long and uses this to anchor itself into the mucosa, causing trauma.

Others just live in the lumen or can penetrate mucosa – *Strongyloides stercoralis*, *Ascaris lumbricoides*, *Enterobius* spp. – retained in the mucosa.

2.5 DEFINITIONS

Microtubules (9+2): The standard arrangement inside a flagellum: 9 pairs of tubes around 2 central ones, like a bundle of straws.

Axoneme: The internal "engine rod" inside a flagellum or cilium that makes it move.

Rhoptries: Club-shaped sacs that inject proteins into the host cell to help the parasite hide and settle in.

Micronemes: Tiny sacs that release glue-like proteins so the parasite can stick to and grip the host cell first.

Conoid: A cone-shaped drill tip at the front of the parasite used to physically pierce the host cell membrane.

Subpellicular microtubules: A skeleton of tubes just under the parasite's skin that keeps its shape and helps it glide into host cells.

Syncytial: A single continuous sheet of cytoplasm with many nuclei but no cell walls between them – the outer skin of tapeworms and flukes is like this.

Oesophageal commissures: The "brain" of nematodes – a nerve ring encircling the oesophagus that coordinates movement and sensation.

Triploblastic acoelomates: Built from three tissue layers but with no body cavity – the inside is solid (e.g. tapeworms, flukes).

Bilaterally symmetrical: Left and right sides are mirror images of each other (like most worms and animals).

FURTHER READING

Field, M. C. (2022). Molecular cellular parasitology: The decades and challenges ahead. *Frontiers in Parasitology*, 1, 963515.

Krüger, T., Schuster, S., & Engstler, M. (2018). Beyond blood: African trypanosomes on the move. *Trends in Parasitology*, 34(12), 1056–1067.

Zuzarte-Luís, V., & Mota, M. M. (2018). Parasite sensing of host nutrients and environmental cues. *Cell Host & Microbe*, 23(6), 749–758. https://doi.org/10.1016/j.chom.2018.05.018

3 Life Cycle of Parasites

The secret of success is constancy of purpose.
Benjamin Disraeli, 1870

CHAPTER OUTLINE

In this chapter, we delve into the intricate life cycles of parasites and explore the stages of development, modes of transmission, and roles of hosts, vectors, and reservoirs. Here's what to expect:

- *Developmental Stages*: Parasites undergo diverse developmental phases, including both sexual and asexual multiplication, within their hosts.
- *Types of Life Cycles*: Learn about direct and indirect life cycles and how they dictate the complexity of parasitic transmission.
- *Host Dynamics*: Understand the distinctions between definitive and intermediate hosts, and their crucial roles in parasite propagation.
- *Vectors and Disease Transmission*: Explore how blood-feeding arthropods serve as vectors, transmitting diseases and perpetuating parasitic cycles.
- *Reservoir Hosts and Zoonosis*: Discover how certain animals act as reservoirs for parasites, leading to zoonotic infections in humans.
- *Modes of Transmission*: From ingestion to skin penetration, uncover the various routes through which parasites are transmitted to humans.
- *Reproduction among Protozoa*: Explore the different forms of reproduction among protozoa, shedding light on their complex life cycles.
- *General Life Cycle of Trematodes*: Delve into the hermaphroditic nature of trematodes and their intricate developmental stages, often involving snails as intermediate hosts.
- *Modes of Infection in Parasitic Trematodes*: Gain insight into the detailed life cycles of parasitic trematodes and their transmission pathways.
- *Generalized Life Cycle of Nematodes*: Understand the four moults during nematode development, and how their life cycles vary in complexity.

DOI: 10.1201/9781003733935-3

- *Intestinal Nematodes*: Explore the characteristics and life cycles of intestinal nematodes, including their impact on human health and longevity.
- *Soil-Transmitted Helminths (Geohelminths)*: Learn about the significance of geohelminths in developing countries, their multiple infection potential, and the three types on the basis of their life cycles.

3.1 GENERAL STAGES OF THE LIFE CYCLE OF PARASITES

Despite the diverse forms of parasites, they all share a common characteristic: An absolute reliance on a host for sustenance and reproduction. This dependence dictates various aspects of the parasite's life cycle, including transmission, invasion, growth, and reproduction.

- The **transmission stage** is where the parasite, in its infectious form, is transmitted from its current host. For example, microscopic liver fluke eggs can cling to blades of grass, waiting for an unsuspecting snail to consume them. Similarly, the larvae of hookworms can burrow through the soles of bare feet to enter a new human host.
- Once inside the host, the parasite enters the **invasion and establishment stage**. During this stage, it uses specialized adaptations to overcome the host's defences and establish itself within the chosen tissue. For instance, tapeworms have hooks that tear through intestinal walls, whereas malaria parasites injected by mosquitoes seek refuge within liver cells. This stage demonstrates the parasite's evolutionary ability to breach the host's defences.
- After establishing itself, the parasite enters the **maturity and reproduction stage.** Here, it thrives and reproduces at a remarkable rate. A single female hookworm can lay up to 200,000 eggs per day, and a liver fluke can produce over 250,000 eggs in its lifetime. This high reproductive capacity ensures parasite survival, even in the context of the host's immune system.
- However, the parasite's story does not end within the host. To complete its life cycle, it must return to the environment **through a dissemination and transmission stage**. For example, tapeworm segments, which carry eggs, are expelled in faeces, while malaria parasites burst out of red blood cells, ready to be taken up by another mosquito. This

stage involves a delicate interaction with the environment, as factors like temperature and humidity affect the parasite's survival and ability to infect.

The complexity of parasite life cycles can vary greatly. Some parasites, such as pinworms, have a relatively straightforward direct cycle and are transmitted directly from host to host through ingested eggs. Others, like the liver fluke, have intricate life cycles that involve multiple hosts and environmental stages. These complex life cycles, developed over millions of years of evolution, ensure the persistence of the parasite and contribute significantly to the ecosystems they inhabit.

All parasites have a series of developmental stages. There may be few or several phases of parasite developmental stages, with at least one stage occurring in the host organism. Developmental phases may involve multiplication. The multiplication phase may be sexual or asexual.

Life cycles may be direct or indirect.

Direct: The parasite requires only one species of host to complete its life cycle, e.g., *E. histolytica* infections in humans.

Indirect: The parasite requires two or more hosts, e.g., filariid worms (both humans/insects).

Host: Can be definitive or intermediate.

- ***Definitive host***: The host in which the parasite reaches sexual maturity and/or undergoes sexual reproduction, e.g., *Schistosoma haematobium* – the definitive host is man. Still, for malaria, the definitive host is the female Anopheles mosquito.
- ***Intermediate host***: These are species of host other than the definitive host that are essential for the completion of life cycles (indirect life cycles). For example, tsetse flies – trypanosomes, *Bulinus truncatus* – schistosomiasis.

Vectors: Apply generally to blood-feeding arthropod intermediate hosts, e.g., mosquitoes, tsetse flies, sandflies, etc., which are transmitters of diseases.

Reservoir host: An organism in which a parasite resides or in which a parasite that infects humans is maintained in the absence of the human host. They are sources of parasites in the environment. They may be mammals, e.g., pigs, cattle, etc., or the environment, e.g., contaminated soil or humans.

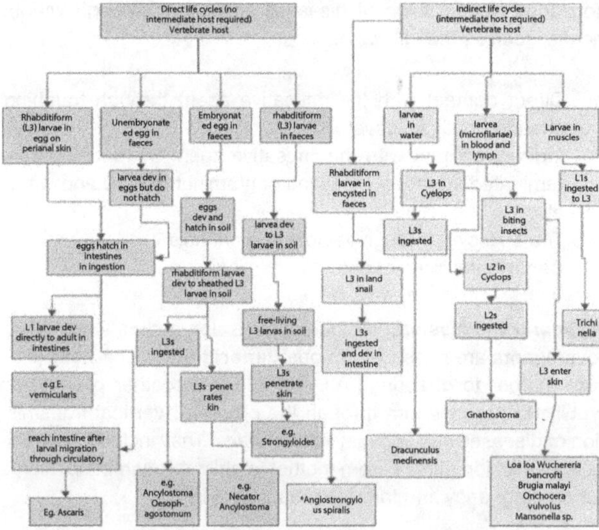

Figure 3.1 Comparison of direct and indirect life cycles of parasitic nematodes. The left panel illustrates a direct life cycle, where transmission occurs via ingestion of or skin penetration by third-stage larvae (L3) from the environment, with examples including *Enterobius vermicularis*, *Ancylostoma* spp., *Oesophagostomum* spp., and *Strongyloides* spp. The right panel depicts an indirect life cycle requiring an intermediate host (e.g., Cyclops), with *Dracunculus medinensis* and *Gnathostoma* spp. shown as examples. L3 = third-stage larvae.

Zoonosis: Parasitic infections in which the normal host is an animal but can produce disease in humans if they become accidentally infected. For example, Leishmaniasis, Chagas, and Trichinellosis/Echinococcosis.

3.2 MODES OF TRANSMISSION OF PARASITIC DISEASES

Horizontal transmission: Refers to the spread of infectious agents (such as parasites, bacteria, viruses, or fungi) from one individual to another within the same generation. For example, contagious diseases such as flu and measles are transmitted horizontally.

Horizontal transmission of diseases can occur through various means, such as the following:

- Direct contact with the causative agent through touching, sharing bodily fluids, etc.
- Indirect contact with the causative agent by touching contaminated surfaces, ingesting contaminated food and water, etc.
- Transmission through vectors and animals
- Behavioural interactions

Vertical transmission: Vertical transmission occurs when infectious agents are passed from one **generation to the next** (e.g., from mother to offspring). An example is a mother passing on syphilis to her newborn through the placenta. Vertical transmission of diseases can occur in several ways. They include congenital transmission, that is, from mother to child through the placenta during pregnancy and through breastfeeding

3.2.1 TRANSMISSION ROUTES OF PARASITES

Parasites can be transmitted through various routes. The infective stages may be transmitted to a person through:

- Ingestion of parasite ova/cyst/oocyst in food/water or hands contaminated with faeces containing the infective form of the parasite (feco-oral) e.g., *Entamoeba histolytica*, *Balantidium coli*, *Giardia lamblia*, *Enterobius vermicularis*, *Trichuris trichiura*.
- Ingestion of parasite in raw or semi-cooked meat, e.g., *Taenia saginata*, *Taenia solium*, *Trichinella spiralis*.
- Ingestion of parasite in raw or uncooked fish, e.g., *Diphyllobothrium latum*.
- Ingestion of parasite in raw or uncooked freshwater crab/crayfish, e.g., *Paragonimus westermani, Fasciolopsis buski*.
- Ingestion of parasite in water containing infected cyclops, e.g., *Dracunculus medinensis*.
- Skin penetration from soil, e.g., hookworms/*Strongyloides stercoralis*.
- Skin penetration through water contact, e.g., *Schistosoma haematobium*, *S. mansoni*, *S. intercalatum*.

- Insect bites (entering through the bites/inoculation through vectors), e.g., *Wuchereria bancrofti*, *Onchocerca volvulus*, *Brugia malayi*, *Loa loa*, *Plasmodia* spp., *Trypanosoma* spp., *Leishmania* spp.
- By sexual contact: e.g., *Trichomonas vaginalis*.
- Infected faeces of an insect vector, e.g., Chagas disease – *Trypanosoma cruzi*.
- Oro-anal practices. *Entamoeba histolytica*, *Cryptosporidium parvum*, and most of the intestinal/diarrhoea-related protozoa.

3.3 DIVERSITY OF HABITATS AND LIFE CYCLES

Life cycle could involve only human hosts, or human-arthropod hosts, or human-wild/game vertebrates, or human vectors, wild/game/domestic vertebrate hosts, etc. Habitat preference could be the lumen, blood, or tissue, in which case the organisms could be lumen, blood, or tissue-dwelling, or they could be intracellular or extracellular organisms.

1. ***Phylogenetic diversity***
   The absence or presence of some essential organelles in some of the organisms. For example, the lack of endoplasmic reticulum, Golgi bodies and mitochondria in *Giardia lamblia*, and the lack of Golgi bodies in *Entamoeba* spp.
2. ***Adaptations to metabolism***
   In some protozoa, adaptation to metabolism might be responsible for the transformation of some facultative forms to obligate lifestyles. The adaptations include:
   a. The absence of some enzyme systems that are obtained from the host organism.
   b. The inability to synthesize lipids de novo.
   c. The inability to synthesize purines and pyrimidines de novo (these are obtained through salvage pathways)
   d. Dependence on the host to supply amino acids.
   e. The use of aerobic metabolism in arthropod vectors and anaerobic metabolism in vertebrate hosts.
   f. The loss of unessential organelles for parasitism, e.g., locomotory organelles, in the Apicomplexa group.
3. ***Presence of specialized surfaces/organelles***
   The body surfaces of protozoans are specialized and may possess organelles modified for:
   a. Attachment (e.g., sucking disc of *Giardia* spp.).

b. Penetration, such as rhoptries of *Apicomplexa*.
c. Adhesion, such as adhesion proteins/lectins of *Entamoeba histolytica*.
d. Nutritional acquisition and evasion from host immune responses.
e. There are also some important internal organelles, such as glycosomes and kinetoplasts, which are found in trypanosomes.

4. ***Presence of specialized cytoskeleton***

   Protozoans have submicrotubules, which give them their unique shape and often help with movement. Protozoans such as amoeba lack microtubules but have actin filaments attached to their plasma membrane.

5. ***Encystation and excystation***

   Endoparasitic protozoa undergo encystation, i.e., they form cysts that are able to survive the harsh external conditions. A typical protozoan cyst is made up of a round mass of protoplasm enveloped in tough walls containing chitin as the major biopolymer. The wall is secreted by the trophozoites during the process of encystment.

   Protozoans can also excyst based on conditions related to pH, the presence of bile salts and variations in CO_2 and O_2 tension in their habitats. Cysts of protozoa have four main functions.

6. ***Mode of reproduction***

   Protozoans undergo different forms of reproduction. Reproduction could be by binary fission, as in *Entamoeba* spp., or conjugation, as in *Balantidium coli*. Protozoans can also undergo multiple types of fission (schizogony or sporogony), which occurs in the *Apicomplexa* group, and sometimes endodyogeny, which can occur in *Toxoplasma* spp.

3.3.1 FORMS OF REPRODUCTION AMONG PROTOZOA

a. ***Binary fission (asexual multiplication)***

   Organisms are divided into two categories (duplication). The plane of division depends on the group/class. The plane of division is random for sarcodina, longitudinal for flagellates, and transverse for ciliates. Nuclear division is mitotic.

b. ***Endodyogeny (asexual)***

   Common in *Toxoplasma gondii* and several related organisms. Two daughter cells form within the parent cell, which then ruptures to release smaller progeny that grow to full size.

c. ***Multiple fission***

I. ***Schizogony (asexual)***

The nucleus of the organism divides repeatedly before the division of the cytoplasm (cytokinesis). Division leads to the production of uni-nucleate daughter cells (merozoites). The cells in which the division occurs are referred to as schizonts.

II. ***Sporogony (sexual)***

Occurs after the fusion of gametes (fertilization). It involves encystation of the zygote to form an oocyst (sporont). The formation of daughter cells is referred to as sporozoites. The cells in which division occurs are referred to as sporocysts.

3.3.2 GENERAL LIFE CYCLE OF PARASITES IN SUB-PHYLUM SARCODINA

The life cycles of sarcodine parasites occur in distinct stages:

- Cysts are transmitted through faeces.
- Upon reaching the gut of the new host, *Entamoeba histolytica* cysts transform into trophozoites, armed with digestive enzymes that enable them to burrow through the intestinal lining.
- Trophozoites divide rapidly, giving rise to cysts that can either remain dormant or re-enter the intestinal cycle to inflict further harm.
- Cysts are expelled through the host's faeces, poised to contaminate water and food sources, awaiting their next unsuspecting host.

While the aforementioned stages serve as a framework, the life cycles of parasites vary significantly within the phylum Sarcodina. Some, like *Entamoeba*, exhibit a straightforward direct life cycle, while others, such as *Naegleria fowleri*, demonstrate intricate indirect life cycles encompassing environmental stages and multiple hosts.

3.3.3 GENERAL LIFE CYCLE OF PARASITES IN SUB-PHYLUM MASTIGOPHORA

- The transmission stage showcases the diverse strategies employed by the parasite for transmission, with some relying

on vectors like insects, while others exploit contaminated water and food sources.
- In the invasion and establishment stage, *Trypanosoma brucei gambiense* uses its flagellum to navigate the host's bloodstream, seeking refuge in the lymph nodes and central nervous system. Once it reaches the gut of the new host, *Giardia lamblia* transforms into trophozoites that possess adhesive discs, enabling them to anchor themselves to the intestinal lining.
- Some parasites undergo binary fission within the bloodstream, releasing daughter cells that perpetuate the infectious cycle. Others rapidly divide, forming cysts that can either remain dormant or re-enter the intestinal cycle to inflict further harm.
- Through the cyclical feeding of the tsetse fly, *Trypanosoma brucei gambiense* completes its complex life cycle, ensuring its perpetuation within the ecosystem. *Giardia lamblia* cysts, packaged for survival, are expelled through the host's faeces, ready to contaminate water sources and perpetuate the cycle of infection.

Within the phylum Mastigophora, some, such as *Trichomonas vaginalis*, possess a straightforward direct life cycle, while others, such as *Leishmania donovani*, exhibit complex indirect life cycles that involve multiple hosts and environmental stages.

3.3.4 GENERAL LIFE CYCLE OF PARASITES IN SUB-PHYLUM CILIOPHORA

- Cysts are transmitted through contaminated food or water.
- *Balantidium coli* cysts, upon reaching the new host's gut, transform into trophozoites equipped with powerful cilia that enable them to swim through the intestinal contents and burrow into the epithelial lining. *Nyctotherus cordiformis* utilizes its cilia to navigate crevices and anchor itself to the intestinal wall.
- *Balantidium coli* undergoes binary fission within the intestinal tract, releasing daughter cells that continue the infectious cycle. *Nyctotherus cordiformis*, within its cellular haven, undergoes conjugation resulting in the release of even more infectious cysts.
- *Balantidium coli* and *Nyctotherus cordiformis* cysts, packaged for survival, are expelled through the host's faeces, ready to contaminate water sources and perpetuate the cycle of infection.

3.3.5 GENERAL LIFE CYCLE OF PARASITES IN SUB-PHYLUM APICOMPLEXA

Apicomplexan parasites, known for their distinctive apical complex, encompass a diverse array of species with varying degrees of complexity. Some, such as the single-celled *Plasmodium falciparum*, embark on a mesmerizing journey through a mosquito and a human host, while others, like the multicellular *Cryptosporidium parvum*, remain confined to the intestinal tract, reproducing within their microscopic dwellings.

- The transmission stage sets the scene, where the parasite, in its infectious form, prepares to depart from its current host and set out on a perilous journey towards a new one. Picture *Plasmodium falciparum* gametocytes, nestled within red blood cells of an infected individual, waiting for their chance encounter with a hungry Anopheles mosquito. Other apicomplexans, such as *Toxoplasma gondii*, release their infectious oocysts directly into the environment, ready to be consumed by unsuspecting herbivores or omnivores. This stage showcases the parasite's diverse strategies for transmission, with some relying on vector-borne routes, while others exploit contaminated food and water sources.
- The second act introduces the invasion and establishment stage, a dramatic display of the parasite's remarkable adaptations. *Plasmodium falciparum* sporozoites, injected by the mosquito, traverse the human bloodstream until they come across liver cells, where they burrow in and initiate a complex replication cycle. *Toxoplasma gondii* oocysts, upon reaching the new host's gut, transform into sporozoites that invade intestinal epithelial cells, establishing a foothold within the host's tissues. This stage highlights the parasite's sophisticated invasive strategies, utilizing specialized structures and enzymes to breach the host's defences and secure a vital haven for growth and reproduction.
- Once it has established its presence, the parasite enters the maturity and reproduction stage, a period of exponential growth and multiplication. *Plasmodium falciparum* undergoes multiple rounds of replication within liver cells and red blood cells, releasing infectious merozoites that continue the cycle within the bloodstream. *Toxoplasma gondii* undergoes both asexual and sexual reproduction within its host cell, releasing oocysts that are shed into the environment, perpetuating the cycle of infection. This stage emphasizes

the parasite's remarkable reproductive capacity, ensuring its continued proliferation and potential for widespread transmission.

- The dissemination and transmission stage marks the parasite's return to the environment, completing its intricate life cycle. *Plasmodium falciparum* gametocytes, formed within red blood cells, are taken up by another Anopheles mosquito during a blood meal, restarting the cycle within the insect vector. *Toxoplasma gondii* oocysts, expelled through the faeces of infected animals, remain dormant in the environment until ingested by a new host, perpetuating the parasite's existence. This stage concludes the parasite's complex performance, showcasing its remarkable adaptations for successful transmission and ensuring its continued survival across generations.

Although the general stages described above serve as a framework, the specific sequence of events in the life cycle of the apicomplexan parasite can vary significantly within the phylum. For example, *Babesia bigemina* follows a relatively straightforward life cycle, whereas *Plasmodium vivax* displays complex dormant stages in the liver, adding another layer of intricacy to their existence. This wide range of variations highlights the incredible adaptability and evolutionary creativity of these captivating parasites.

3.3.6 GENERAL LIFE CYCLE OF PARASITES IN CLASS TREMATODA

Trematode parasites are easily recognized by their flat bodies and specialized suckers used for attachment. They encompass a wide range of species with varying levels of complexity.

- The transmission stage is when the parasite, in its infectious form, prepares to leave its current host and embark on a perilous journey towards a new one. The tiny eggs of *Fasciola hepatica*, nestled among the waste of sheep or cattle, patiently await their chance encounter with an unsuspecting snail. Other trematodes, such as *Schistosoma mansoni*, release their infectious cercariae directly into freshwater bodies, ready to penetrate the skin of a human host.
- Once the *Fasciola hepatica* eggs reach the new host's gut, they hatch into miracidia that burrow through the intestinal wall and begin a complex migration through the bloodstream

and various organs. Eventually, in the liver, they mature into adults and start laying eggs to continue the cycle. *Schistosoma mansoni* cercariae, upon penetrating the human skin, transform into schistosomula that migrate through the bloodstream and eventually settle in the blood vessels of the urinary tract or intestines.

- After establishing their presence, the parasites move on to the stage of maturity and reproduction, which is a period of exponential growth and multiplication. The adult *Fasciola hepatica* within the liver lays thousands of eggs that are expelled through the host's bile ducts and eventually reach

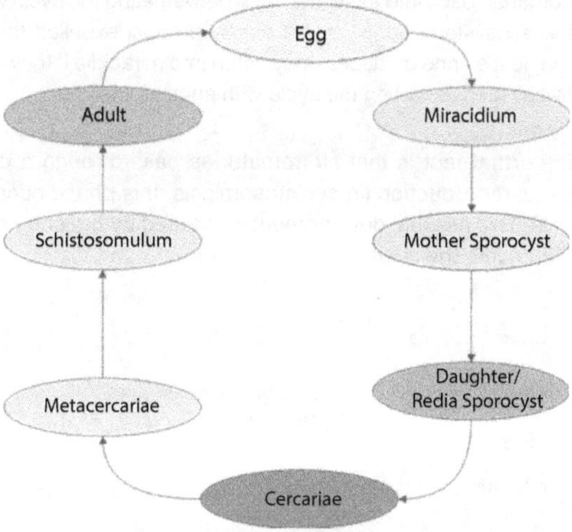

Figure 3.2 Generalized life cycle stages of a digenetic trematode (fluke). The cycle begins with eggs, which release free-swimming miracidia. Miracidia infect an intermediate host (typically a snail), where they develop into mother sporocysts, followed by daughter sporocysts or rediae. These produce cercariae (not shown), which may encyst as metacercariae in a second intermediate host or environment. After ingestion by the definitive host, metacercariae excyst into schistosomula (or juvenile flukes) and mature into adult worms. (Stages vary by species; e.g., in *Schistosoma* spp., cercariae directly penetrate skin as schistosomula without metacercarial encystment.)

the environment, initiating the cycle once again. *Schistosoma mansoni* pairs mate within the blood vessels, releasing eggs that either trigger inflammation and tissue damage within the host or are expelled through urine or faeces, depending on the species. This stage highlights the remarkable reproductive capacity of the parasite, ensuring its continued proliferation and potential for widespread transmission.

- The final stage, known as the dissemination and transmission phase, marks the parasite's return to the environment, completing its intricate life cycle. The *Fasciola hepatica* eggs are expelled through the host's faeces and are ingested by snails, where they undergo further development and release infectious cercariae back into the water, thus perpetuating the cycle within the ecosystem. *Schistosoma mansoni* eggs, expelled through the host's urine or faeces, may hatch into miracidia if they reach freshwater, restarting the cycle with another snail host.

One important fact is that all trematodes pass through a phase of asexual reproduction (in schistosomiasis, this phase occurs in the snail). This asexual development is initiated by the entry of the miracidium into the snail.

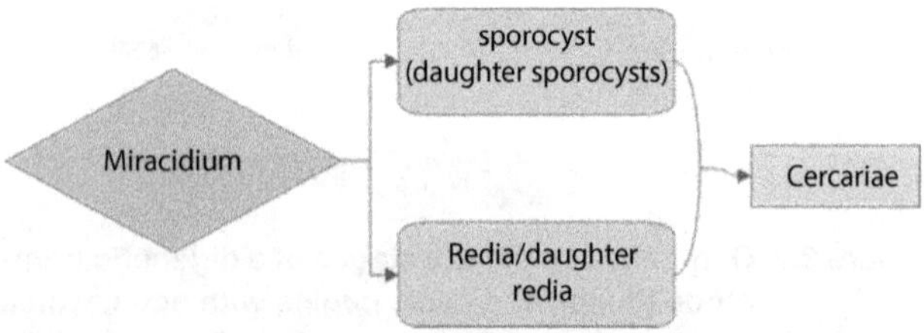

Figure 3.3 Larval developmental stages of a trematode within the intermediate snail host. The free-swimming miracidium penetrates the snail and transforms into a sporocyst. The sporocyst produces either daughter sporocysts or rediae (including daughter rediae), which in turn generate cercariae. Cercariae are released from the snail to continue the life cycle.

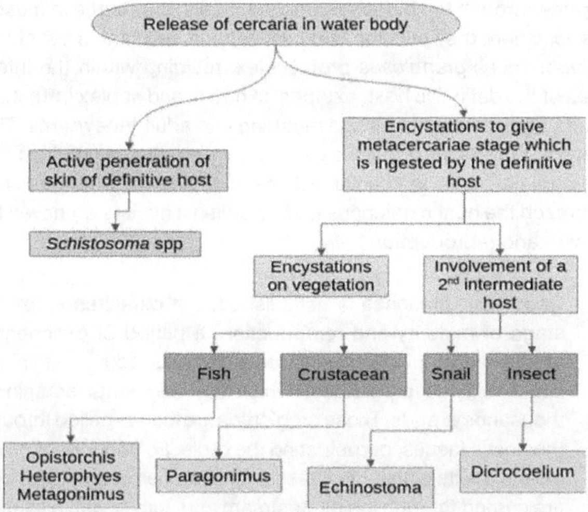

Figure 3.4 Mode of Infection in Parasitic Trematodes.

3.3.7 GENERAL LIFE CYCLE OF PARASITES CLASS CESTODA

The Cestoda phylum, commonly known as tapeworms, is characterized by their ribbon-like shapes and intricate life cycles. Cestode parasites possess segmented bodies and specialized hooks for attachment, encompassing a wide range of species with varying complexities.

- During the transmission stage, the parasite, in its infectious form, prepares to leave its current host and embark on a journey towards a new one. Microscopic *Taenia saginata* eggs, nestled among the debris of human faeces, patiently await their opportunity to encounter an unsuspecting herbivore. Other cestodes, such as *Echinococcus granulosus*, release their infectious scolex-bearing protoscolex within the tissues of their intermediate host, ready to be ingested by a definitive host. This stage demonstrates the diverse strategies employed by the parasite for transmission, some relying on contaminated water and food sources, while others utilize the dynamics of the food chain within their ecosystem.

The second act showcases the remarkable adaptability of the parasite. *Taenia saginata* eggs, upon reaching the gut of the new host, hatch into oncospheres that tunnel through the intestinal wall and migrate through the bloodstream. Eventually, they settle in muscle tissue, where they develop into cysticerci, a dormant larval stage. *Echinococcus granulosus* protoscolex, residing within the intestines of the definitive host, extends its hooks and scolex, attaching itself to the intestinal wall and maturing into adult tapeworms. This stage highlights the sophisticated invasive strategies employed by the parasite, utilizing specialized enzymes and migratory abilities to breach the host's defences and establish a necessary haven for growth and reproduction.

- Once their presence is established, the parasites enter the stage of maturity and reproduction, a period of exponential growth and multiplication. *Taenia saginata* adults within the intestine shed proglottids, which are segments containing thousands of eggs. These proglottids are then expelled through the host's faeces, perpetuating the cycle. *Echinococcus granulosus* adults within the intestine produce protoscolex, which are carried through the bloodstream and encyst within various organs, patiently awaiting another definitive host to continue the cycle. This stage emphasizes the remarkable reproductive ability of the parasite, ensuring its continuous proliferation and potential for widespread transmission.
- The final act, the stage of dissemination and transmission, marks the parasite's return to the environment, completing its intricate life cycle. *Taenia saginata* eggs, which are expelled through faeces, are ingested by herbivores, where they develop into cysticerci, closing the loop within the ecosystem. *Echinococcus granulosus* cysts within the organs of the definitive host are ingested by another definitive host, releasing protoscolex within the new intestine and restarting the cycle. This stage concludes the complex performance of the parasite, showcasing their remarkable adaptations for successful transmission and ensuring their continued survival across generations.

3.3.8 GENERALIZED PSEUDOPHYLLIDEAN LIFE CYCLE

- Their eggs contain immature embryos when discharged.
- Their eggs are discharged in stool.
- Their embryos develop, become ciliated, and are called coracidia (larvae), which are aquatic in nature.
- Their larvae have six hooks (hexacanth larvae).
- Because larvae are spherical in shape, it is also referred to as the oncosphere.

- Coracidium swims in water and is usually ingested by a first intermediate host (copepod-arthropod).
- Within the copepod, it is transformed into a procercoid larva.
- When the copepod is fed on by the appropriate fish, the procercoids are released to infect the muscles of the fish. They are then transformed into the plerocercoid larvae (infective stage to humans).

In eggs in water (coracidium) → copepods
In copepods (procercoid) → fish
In fish (plerocercoid) → man

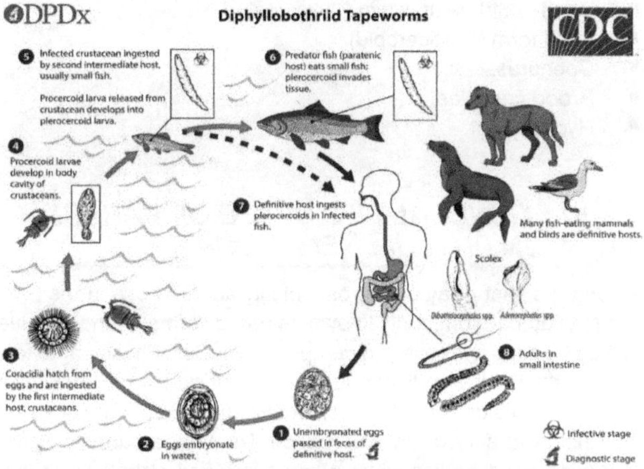

Figure 3.5 Life cycle of diphyllobothriid tapeworms (broad fish tapeworms). Unembryonated eggs (1) are passed in the faeces of the definitive host and embryonate in water (2). Coracidia hatch from eggs and are ingested by the first intermediate host, crustaceans (3). Within the crustacean, the coracidium develops into a procercoid larva, which then matures into a plerocercoid larva in the body cavity (4). An infected crustacean is ingested by a second intermediate host, usually a small fish, where the plerocercoid larva develops further (5). A predator fish (paratenic host) may eat the small fish, with the plerocercoid invading tissues (6). The definitive host (e.g., fish-eating mammal or bird) becomes infected by ingesting plerocercoids in infected fish (7). Adults reside in the small intestine (8), completing the cycle.

3.3.9 GENERALIZED CYCLOPHYLLIDEAN LIFE CYCLE

- Eggs develop into hexacanth larvae (oncospheres).
- The oncosphere is eaten by the intermediate host.
- Larvae enter the circulatory system of the intermediate host and are carried to other parts of the body.
- Eggs may also be picked up by arthropods, which may be eaten by, e.g., birds, and these larvae may end up in the tissues of the birds (abnormal hosts).
- Within the tissues, larvae develop into one of several forms.
- Bladder worm (Cysticercus).
- Head could be out – evaginated.
- Head could be drawn in – invaginated.
- Solid form (Cysticercoid).
- Coenurus.
- Brood capsules.
- Hydatid cyst.

3.3.10 GENERAL LIFE CYCLE OF PARASITES IN PHYLUM NEMATODA

Among the vast array of microscopic invaders, those in the phylum Nematoda, commonly known as roundworms, stand out due to their twisting journeys and complex life cycles. These parasites, such as the hookworms that burrow into our skin or the *Trichinella spiralis* that reside in our tissues, create intricate connections with their hosts to survive and reproduce. Nematode parasites possess elongated bodies without segments and strong outer layers, and they encompass a diverse range of species with varying degrees of complexity.

- The transmission stage commences, during which the parasite, in its infectious form, prepares to depart from its current host and venture towards a new one. Tiny *Ascaris lumbricoides* eggs, nestled among human faecal matter, patiently await unsuspecting hosts to cross their path. Other nematodes, such as *Trichinella spiralis*, release their infectious larvae directly into the muscle tissue of infected animals, and are ready to be consumed by a new predator. This stage highlights the diverse strategies employed by parasites for transmission, some relying on contaminated water and food sources, whereas others take advantage of the dynamics of the food chain within their ecosystem.

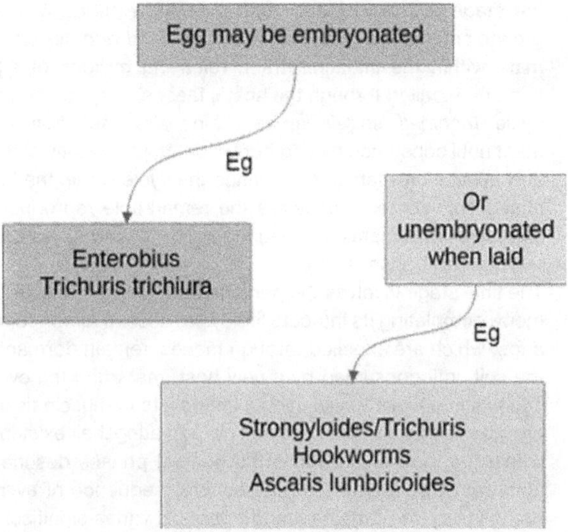

Figure 3.6 Comparison of nematode egg morphology at the time of oviposition. Some nematode eggs are embryonated (fully developed containing a larva) when laid by the female, as seen in *Enterobius* and *Trichuris trichiura*. Other nematode eggs are unembryonated when laid and require a period of development in the external environment before becoming infective, as seen in hookworms, Strongyloides, and *Ascaris lumbricoides*.

The second phase introduces the stage of invasion and establishment, demonstrating the parasite's incredible adaptability. Upon reaching the digestive system of the new host, *Ascaris lumbricoides* eggs hatch into larvae that burrow through the intestinal wall and embark on an exhilarating journey through the bloodstream. Eventually, they reach the lungs, where they are coughed up, migrate to the small intestine, and finally mature into adult worms. *Trichinella spiralis* larvae, within the muscle tissue of the new host, encase themselves in cysts and patiently await their chance to continue the cycle within another predator. This stage highlights the parasite's sophisticated invasive strategies, utilizing specialized enzymes and burrowing abilities to penetrate the host's defences and establish a crucial haven for growth and reproduction.

- Once they have established themselves, the parasites enter the stage of maturity and reproduction, a period of rapid growth and multiplication. Adult *Ascaris lumbricoides* worms mate within the intestinal tract, releasing millions of eggs that are expelled through the host's faeces, perpetuating the cycle. *Trichinella spiralis* larvae within their cysts remain dormant until consumed by another predator, where they mature and release new larvae to continue the cycle within the food chain. This stage emphasizes the remarkable reproductive capacity of the parasite, ensuring its continued spread and widespread transmission.
- The final stage involves the parasite returning to the environment, completing its intricate life cycle. *Ascaris lumbricoides* eggs, which are expelled through faeces, remain dormant in the soil until consumed by a new host, restarting the cycle. *Trichinella spiralis* larvae, within their cysts in muscle tissue, are ingested by another predator, perpetuating their existence within the food chain. While the general phases described above provide a structure, the specific sequence of events in the life cycle of the nematode parasite varies significantly within the phylum. Certain parasites, such as pinworms, have a relatively straightforward direct life cycle, while others, like filarial worms, have complex indirect life cycles involving intermediate hosts and environmental stages.

Usually there are four moults during development from ovum to adult and in most species, the third stage larval is the infective stage, but the other larval stages could also be infective.

Worm	Infective Stages	Mode
Enterobius vermicularis	L1 larvae (rhabditiform)	ingested (in eggs)
Ascaris lumbricoides	L2 larvae (rhabditiform)	ingested (in eggs)
Strongyloides	L3 larvae (filariform)	penetrate skin
Necator americanus	L3 larvae (filariform)	penetrate skin
Ancylostoma duodenale	L3 larvae (filariform)	ingested eggs/ penetrate. skin
Onchocerca vulvolus	L3 larvae (filariform)	inoculated by Simulium fly

Worm	Infective Stages	Mode
Wuchereria bancrofti	L3 larvae (filariform)	inoculated by Anopheles
Brugia malayi	L3 larvae (filariform)	inoculated by Mansonia fly
Loa loa	L3 larvae (filariform)	inoculated by Chrysops fly
Mansonella ozzardi	L3 larvae (filariform)	inoculated by Culicoides fly
Dracunculus medinensis	L3 larvae (filariform)	ingestion of infected Cyclops
Trichenella spiralis	L1 larvae (rhabditiform)	ingestion in infected meat

During this process, the outer cuticle is shed four times through ecdysis.

3.4 SERIES OF LARVAL STAGES

- First is the rhabditiform larvae. Larval development is by moulting/growing.
- Second stage larvae rhabditiform – shape of oesophagus (oesophagus is double bulbed). They are particulate feeders when free-living.
- Third stage is the filariform – they have a flat oesophagus

There is an adolescent form that moults to become an adult (juveniles)

- First stage Larva + Moult 1 = Rhabditiform
- Second stage Larva + Moult 2 = Filariform, e.g., hookworms, *Strongyloides* spp.
- Third stage Larva + Moult 3 = Adolescent + Moult 4 = Adult (juvenile)

3.4.1 LIFE CYCLE

Direct: This is common among *Enterobius vermicularis* and *Trichuris trichiura*; the infective larvae moult in the intestine and also among hookworms, *Ascaris lumbricoides* and *Strongyloides stercoralis*.

Indirect: This is common among the blood-associated forms, e.g., filarial worms. The life cycle of hookworms, *Ascaris lumbricoides* and *Strongyloides stercoralis* follows the following pattern.

3.4.1.1 Intestinal Nematodes

- They are roundworms, unsegmented with bilateral symmetry.
- They have a fully functional digestive tract.
- They are long and cylindrical.
- They are dioecious (separate sexes).
- They are dimorphic (males are smaller than females).
- Their egg production varies from few in a day (Strongyloides) to over 200,000 per female per day in Ascaris.
- They have five successive stages in their life cycle (four larval stages and one adult stage).

Egg → L1M1 → L2M2 → L3M3 → L4M4 → Juvenile worm

L = Larval stage M = Moult L4= Adolescent stage

Infective larvae hatch in intestines/soil

↓

penetrate the intestinal wall/skin

↓

gain access into the venules and lymphatics.

↓

enter the circulatory system

↓

move into the right side of the heart.

↓

gain access into the lungs.

↓

then to the bronchioles

↓

to the trachea

then are swallowed into the intestines

3.4.1.2 Soil-Transmitted Helminths (Geohelminths)

Geohelminths are of great importance in the health of many populations in developing countries because the frequency of infection is a general indication of the local level of development, hygiene, and sanitation. Multiple infections usually occur.

Geohelminths are divided into three types according to their life cycle.

3.4.1.2.1 TYPE 1

In type 1, the eggs passed are **embryonated**.

These eggs hatch and reinfect within 2–3 hours, usually through the faecal–oral route.

The eggs do not usually reach the soil, and whenever they do, they do not require any period of development.

e.g., 1. *Enterobius vermicularis* (pinworm).

2. *Trichuris trichiura* (whipworm).

3.4.1.2.2 TYPE 2

In type 2, eggs passed in stool undergo a period of development in the soil before being ingested. Thus, the larvae are released in the stomach.

The larvae can penetrate the mucous membrane of the stomach; they then enter the circulatory system to reach the lungs and pass up the respiratory tract. From the respiratory tract, they enter the oesophagus, then the intestines, where they grow and become adults.

e.g., *Ascaris lumbricoides*

(Figure 3.7)

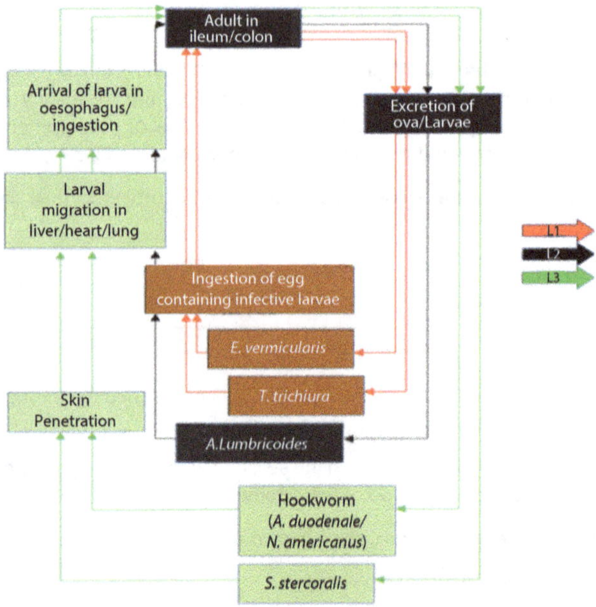

Figure 3.7 **Comparative life cycle pathways of common intestinal nematodes. Adults reside in the ileum or colon and release ova or larvae via feces. Transmission occurs via two main routes: (1) ingestion of eggs containing infective larvae (*Enterobius vermicularis, Trichuris trichiura, Ascaris lumbricoides*), or (2) skin penetration by larvae (hookworms (*Ancylostoma duodenale/ Necator americanus*), Strongyloides stercoralis). Following ingestion or skin penetration, larvae undergo migration through the liver, heart, and lungs before being transported to the oesophagus and subsequently reaching the gestational tissues or intestine, where they mature into adults.**

3.4.1.2.3 TYPE 3

In type 3, the eggs are passed in stool into the soil, where they hatch into larvae and undergo further development before penetration of the skin.

e.g., 1. *Strongyloides stercoralis*

2. *Ancylostoma duodenale*

3. *Necator americanus*

FURTHER READING

Anderson, O. R. (1988). The Flagellates (Phylum: Sarcomastigophora; Subphylum: Mastigophora). *Comparative Protozoology*, 16–34. https://doi.org/10.1007/978-3-662-11340-0_2

Ascaris lumbricoides- Life cycle, Pathogenicity, Clinical Manifestation. (n.d.). Retrieved 13 November 2023, from https://microbenotes.com/ascaris-lumbricoides-life-cycle-pathogenicity-clinical-manifestation/

Brooker, S. & Bundy, D. (2014). Soil-transmitted Helminths (Geohelminths). *Manson's Tropical Diseases*, 1515–1548. https://doi.org/10.1016/B978-0-7020-5101-2.00056-X.

Dey, S., Mohapatra, S., Khokhar, M., Hassan, S., & Pandey, R. K. (2024). Extracellular vesicles in Malaria: Shedding light on pathogenic depths. *ACS Infectious Diseases*, 10(3), 827–844.

Gang, S. S., & Hallem, E. A. (2016). Mechanisms of host seeking by parasitic nematodes. *Molecular and Biochemical Parasitology*, 208(1), 23–32. https://doi.org/10.1016/j.molbiopara.2016.05.007

Hicks, S. J., Theodoropoulos, G., Carrington, S. D., & Corfield, A. P. (2000). The role of mucins in host-parasite interactions. Part I – Protozoan parasites. *Parasitology Today*, 16(11), 476–481. https://doi.org/10.1016/S0169-4758(00)01773-7

Świdersk, Z. & Georgiev, B. (2008). Fundamentals of Cestodology. Volume 14. Aploparaksidae of wild and domesticated birds, by S.K. Bondarenko and V.L. Kontrimavichus (Ed. S.O. Movsesyan). Published by NAUKA, Moscow, 2006. *Acta Parasitologica*, 53(1), 115–116. https://doi.org/10.2478/s11686-008-0014-y

Thibeaux, R., Weber, C., Hon, C. C., Dillies, M. A., Avé, P., Coppée, J. Y., Labruyère, E., & Guillén, N. (2013). Identification of the virulence landscape essential for entamoeba histolytica invasion of the human colon. *PLoS Pathogens*, 9(12), e1003824. https://doi.org/10.1371/JOURNAL.PPAT.1003824

Valigurová, A. & Florent, I. (2021). Nutrient acquisition and attachment strategies in basal lineages: A tough nut to crack in the evolutionary puzzle of apicomplexa. *Microorganisms*, 9(7), 1430. https://doi.org/10.3390/MICROORGANISMS9071430

Verner, Z., Žárský, V., Le, T., Narayanasamy, R. K., Rada, P., Rozbeský, D., Makki, A., Belišová, D., Hrdý, I., Vancová, M., Lender, C., König, C., Bruchhaus, I., & Tachezy, J. (2021). Anaerobic peroxisomes in Entamoeba histolytica metabolise myo-inositol. *PLoS Pathogens*, 17(11), e1010041. https://doi.org/10.1371/JOURNAL.PPAT.1010041

4 Physiology and Biochemistry of Parasites

CHAPTER OUTLINE

In this chapter, we delve into parasite physiology and biochemistry, shedding light on the fundamental processes that govern their survival and interaction with their hosts. Here's what to expect:

- *Host–Parasite Interrelationships*: Explore the dynamic interplay between hosts and parasites, understanding how parasites adapt to their hosts' internal environments for survival.
- *Nutritional Requirements*: Learn about the diverse nutritional needs of parasites, from holozoic feeding mechanisms to the manipulation of host digestive processes.
- *Metabolic Pathways*: Unravel the metabolic intricacies of parasites, including glycolysis, Krebs cycle adaptations, and unique energy production strategies.
- *Environmental Adaptations*: Understand how parasites navigate varying oxygen levels and nutrient availability in different host environments.
- *Current Antiparasitic Drugs and Targets*: Discover the arsenal of drugs targeting essential parasite enzymes, microtubules, membranes, and signalling pathways, and learn about emerging strategies to combat drug resistance.
- *Future Perspectives*: Peek into the future of antiparasitic research, from vaccine development to gene editing and immunomodulation, promising new avenues in parasite control and prevention.

4.1 HOST–PARASITE INTERRELATIONSHIPS

Physiology and biochemistry are very essential for understanding:

- Host–parasite interrelationships.
- Host/agent/environment interactions.

DOI: 10.1201/9781003733935-4

- Host forms the internal environment/habitat needed for the survival/growth/development of the agent.
- To maintain an equilibrium, we need to understand the factors involved, e.g., nutrition/oxygen requirements/growth requirements, etc.

Nutrition of all parasites is holozoic (i.e., they require organic materials particulate/in solution).

Amoebae engulf food particles or droplets through the formation of food vacuoles, and waste products are ejected.

- Many protozoan parasites have permanent mouths (cytostomes or micro-pores) that are used for the ingestion of food.
- Others use pinocytosis (a method of ingesting nutrient materials by drawing fluid through small openings in the body walls
- Protozoan metabolic pathways are similar to those of higher animals and require the same type of organic/inorganic compounds.
- Metabolic pathways play an essential role in the design of antiparasitic drugs/compounds to block these pathways, e.g., the sulphate drugs used in malaria to block the folate synthesis.
- Some intestinal parasites can significantly interfere with the digestion/absorption and affect the nutritional status of their hosts, e.g., *Giardia* and *Cryptosporidium*.
- Some protozoa destroy host cells/tissues due to their metabolic activities. This tends to increase host nutritional needs.
- Extra/intra-cellular parasites that destroy cells while feeding can lead to organ dysfunction and serious life-threatening consequences.

The nature of parasitism leads to different degrees of metabolic dependence on the host.

Metabolic/physiological dependence includes the need for:

- Developmental stimuli
- Nutritional materials
- Digestive enzymes
- Control of maturation/mitosis

Developmental stimuli: Refers to stimuli that trigger the parasite to enter/move to the next developmental stage. By these stimuli, the parasite recognizes the environment has become hostile, and it then moves to the next phase of its development. Parasites respond to some factors/parameters in their environment (create some awareness).

E.g., Metacercaria of trematodes, oocysts of Apicomplexa, infective larvae of nematodes: The above examples utilize the high pCO_2 of the intestines as a signal for encystation or ensheathment. These activities are greatly enhanced by the redox potential (Eh) of the presence of bile. On the contrary, cestodes use bile as a signal for evagination of their scolices for attachment. Other factors include body temperature/body chemistry, etc.

Nutritional dependence: This differs in that there is dependence on digested/undigested food of the host, blood/fluids/tissues of the host, and secretions/enzymes of the host. In some cases, one host can satisfy the needs of the parasite; in others, however, more than one host is needed.

In cases where more than one host is required, different developmental stages tend to occur in different hosts, e.g., *Schistosoma haematobium* in the mesenteric veins of humans is 100% dependent on the host for food and oxygen.

Digestive enzymes: Enzymes are needed to digest food from the host, e.g., trematodes/nematodes have enzymes that hydrolyse complex molecules, but cestodes that take their food by absorption need already digested food (carbohydrates/fats/proteins). They normally utilize the host's enzymes. It is worth noting that some larval cestodes can digest their own food.

Some parasites have lost the enzymes needed for certain fundamental processes, e.g., cestodes cannot digest lipids de novo and as such depend on the host. In some instances, the host can utilize the parasite's system for digestion (two-way benefit), e.g., Plerocercoids (spagana) of Spirometra release substances (growth factors) which induce an increase in the growth weight of the infected host.

Other factors like control of maturation influence some parasites' dependence on the host for maturation/developmental processes in the following ways:

- Usually, the endocrine system of the host stimulates the metabolic process of the parasite.
- There is synchronization of the reproductive phases of the intermediate host/parasite to the benefit of the parasite.

For those parasites that are transmitted by vectors, these phases may also coincide with the natural occurrence of the vectors. Hormonal activities of the host can influence the life cycle of the parasites. These life cycles synchronize with that of their host and may involve the release of eggs/ova/cysts, etc. to infect the susceptible host. There are circadian rhythms in host–parasite relationships where the release of parasites (infective forms) is known to synchronize with the presence or activity of the susceptible host. It is known that the maturation of some parasites is related to the levels of hormones in the host.

4.1.1 PROTOZOA

Protozoans vary in relation to their physiology and resistance, in that while some ingest particulate food, others feed by osmosis. Food particles or substances are surrounded by fluid and circulate in the endoplasm (food vacuole). Some integral factors surrounding the physiology and resistance structures and mechanisms of protozoans include:

- During circulation, digestive enzymes/substances are secreted into the food vacuoles.
- Substances digested vary widely; e.g., *E. histolytica*, the substances dissolved include tissue cells, etc.
- After digestion–absorption is through the body walls, cytoplasm, and cytophage.
- Reserves of food may be stored as glycogen, fats, oils, etc.
- Food/growth requirements.
- Many parasitic protozoa store food in the form of metachromatids (because they stain like chromatin) granules.
- When protozoan parasites are about to encyst, amoebic organisms form chromatid bodies (the chromatid bodies contain stores of food substances).

4.1.1.1 Sub-phylum Sarcodina (Amoebae)

- They are particulate feeders.
- They lack mitochondria/hydrogenases (organelles that produce molecular hydrogen as the main metabolic product) and a functional Krebs cycle.
- Carbohydrate is utilized as the main source of food, and it is absorbed as glucose.

- Carbohydrate in the form of starch, e.g., rice starch, has been found to support their growth.
- Energy is obtained by glycolytic phosphorylation through the Embden–Meyerhof pathway.
- Lactose is not an end product of digestion because it lacks lactose dehydrogenase.
- Pyruvate is converted to ethanol and carbon dioxide, which are the main end products of anaerobic metabolism.
- Protein metabolism is not well understood, but the presence of proteolytic enzymes (protease/collagen, etc.) has been detected, e.g., cysteine proteinase.
- Their nitrogen requirements are based on only amino acids and other nitrogenous compounds of low molecular weight.

4.1.1.2 Sub-phylum Mastigophora (Flagellates)

- They are particulate feeders.
- Intestinal forms feed on detritus/bacteria/yeast.
- Buccal and vaginal forms feed on leukocytes.
- *Trichomonas vaginalis* and *Giardia lamblia* lack mitochondria like *E. histolytica*; however, *Trichomonas vaginalis* contains hydrogenases which constitute separate compartments of energy metabolism, e.g.. paracostal and paraxostylar bodies.
- *Giardia lamblia* contains a lysosome-like organelle. All enzyme activities of *Giardia lamblia* take place in the cytosol.
- Carbohydrates are the main source of energy, and metabolism is fermentative in the intestinal forms.
- Parasitic forms utilize simpler forms of carbohydrates, e.g., hexose/amino acids/fats.
- Glucose metabolism utilizes the E–M pathway to give pyruvate.
- Glycolysis in *Trichomonas vaginalis* gives rise to glycerol/lactate/carbon dioxide and hydrogen.
- In both *Trichomonas vaginalis* and *Giardia lamblia*, pyruvate can further be metabolized to give acetyl-CoA.
- Little is known about amino acid and protein metabolism.
- *Trichomonas vaginalis* requires fatty acids and cholesterol as essential nutrients.
- The blood forms, e.g., trypanosome and *Leishmania* parasites undergo metabolic switches in the host bloodstream as well as that of the vectors.

- Trypanosome vectors and *Leishmania* parasites possess glycosomes/trypanothione (organelles) which play essential roles in protecting the organisms against oxidative stress.
- Glycosomes are known to contain at least nine enzymes needed in the glycolytic pathway.
- Glycosomes also play major roles in carbon dioxide fixation/pyrimidine biosynthesis/oxidation of fatty acids/biosynthesis of lipids and purine salvage.
- Trypanothione plays a significant role in the maintenance of a correct redox potential in trypanosomastids.

In bloodstream forms

- Trypomastigote forms of *Trypanosoma brucei* possess no energy stores and cannot oxidize amino acids/fatty acids and so are entirely dependent on exogenous supply of carbohydrates (glucose/fructose/mannose or glycerol) for energy.
- Aerobic glycolysis occurs through the E–M pathway using enzymes in the glycosomes/mitochondria/cytosol.
- End products of carbohydrate metabolism are pyruvate/traces of carbon dioxide and glycerol.
- Most blood forms cannot further metabolize pyruvate; however, under anaerobic conditions, long/slender bloodstream forms can utilize glucose, which is metabolized into pyruvate and glycerol.
- Procystic (vector) forms undergo metabolic switches using their kinetoplasts.

4.1.1.3 Sub-phylum Apicomplexa

- Plasmodium parasites lack carbohydrate reserves.
- The primary source of energy is glucose from the blood.
- They can oxidize various carbohydrate forms including fructose/maltose and glucose.
- Glucose is the only support for growth and reproduction.
- Plasmodia parasites do not oxidize glucose completely to carbon dioxide and water.
- Enzymes of typical glycolytic pathways are known to be present in plasmodia parasites, suggesting the release of unusable energy as ATP.
- The malaria parasite is known to be extremely wasteful in its energy production pathway. It uses more than it produces. Usually, there is accumulation of lactic acid.

- If the accumulation is not neutralized the reproduction process of the parasite is affected.
- In the rings forms (trophozoites), the glucose consumption is very low.
- All plasmodia parasites are capable of fixing carbon dioxide.
- Some stages can produce lipids, but they lack storage reserves.
- Proteins are synthesized using carbon from carbon dioxide fixation, free amino acids from plasma or blood cells, and proteolysis of haemoglobin (Hb).
- *P. burgi* is known to ingest Hb from the cytoplasm of the host RBCs in molecules or groups of molecules.
- It has been found that malaria parasites can split Hb into haem and globin.
- It is estimated that 76% of Hb in infected RBCs is destroyed during the life of the parasite.
- Hematin (pigment produced from Hb breakdown) is not utilized by the parasite but is rather released as a characteristic malaria pigment.

4.1.1.4 Sub-phylum Ciliophora (Ciliates)

- Require starch for growth.
- Oxygen requirements.
- Oxygen requirements differ. There are two groups.
- Aerobic requires oxygen.
- Anaerobic organisms require no oxygen.
- Some anaerobic species, being obligate, cannot utilize oxygen at all; little oxygen could be very toxic.
- Other facultative ones could survive in the presence of traces of oxygen.

4.1.1.5 Sub-phylum Mastigophora (Flagellates)

- It is not clear whether they are true obligate anaerobes.
- Research shows that *Trichomonas* requires little or no oxygen for development due to the location in the body of their hosts.
- Some Trypanosomes are facultative while some *Leishmania* parasites are known to be aerobes.

4.1.1.6 Sub-phylum Sarcodina (Amoebae)

- *E. histolytica* could be facultative or anaerobic.
- They grow best in complete absence of oxygen or with just traces of oxygen. An increase in oxygen is very toxic.
- They proliferate at low oxidation/reduction (redox) Eh potentials.
- Some Acanthamoeba may be strictly aerobic.

4.1.1.7 Sub-phylum Apicomplexa

- All the intracellular forms, e.g., Plasmodia are aerobic.
- This is because the blooaerobic.ch in oxygen.
- Intestinal flagellates, however, require little or no oxygen for their development.

4.1.1.8 Sub-phylum Ciliophora (Ciliates)

- The oxygen requirement of endoparasitic ciliates varies among the species and their location.
- It is assumed that in this group there are both aerobes and anaerobes.
- *Balantidium coli* is known to utilize oxygen.

4.1.2 METAZOA

4.1.2.1 Phylum Platyhelminthes (Flatworm)

4.1.2.1.1 SUB-PHYLUM TREMATODA (FLUKES)

4.1.2.1.1.1 Nutritional and Growth Requirements

- They are suctorial feeders. They show little variation in feeding mechanism.
- They feed mainly on semi-fluids and soft host tissue.
- Most suck food using suckers/pharynx.
- Tegument has considerable absorption potential.
- Tegument is used for the absorption of food.
- E.g., Schistosomes can take carbohydrates (fructose, mannose/glucosamine, ribose), amino acids (methionine, glutamate, glycine, arginine, alanine, tryptophan), and pyrimidines (cytosine, thymidine, and uracil) through their tegument.

- Food can also be taken by different transport mechanisms, i.e., diffusion/active transport/mediated transport/facilitated, etc.
- *S. mansoni* takes, among other things, blood through the tegument,
- Food can also be digested in the lumen of the intestines using several digestive enzymes,
- There is also "placental" digestion – certain adhesive organs, which are usually used for attachment, serve under some conditions as extra corporeal organs of digestion, e.g., hold-fasts are known to be both digestive and "placental."
- Adult trematodes utilize carbohydrate as a primary source of energy.
- Glucose is usually absorbed and converted to glycogen.
- Metabolism is predominantly anaerobic.
- Some trematodes, e.g., Fasciola, are known to move from aerobic digestion to anaerobic digestion processes as they grow juveniles to adults.
- Glucose metabolism is more efficient in some female trematodes than in males.
- In trematodes, amino acid absorption appears to occur through the tegument, just as in the case of carbohydrate uptake.
- Similarly, uptake of proteins is through a mixture of mediated/diffusion transports.
- There are specific/localized sites of amino acid transport.
- Amino acids play a significant role as a source of energy in blood feeders.
- Trematodes are not able to synthesize long chain fatty acids/lipids de novo.
- Trematodes acquire lipids exogenously from fluids, tissues, and cell membranes of the host.

4.1.2.1.2 CLASS CESTODA (TAPEWORMS)

The physiology/biochemistry of Cestodes is unique due to

- Their unusual location/habitat (environment)
- Their basic morphology
- Growth of their strobila

4.1.2.1.2.1 Environment

- Physiological properties change constantly.
- Nutritional levels vary in relation to feeding patterns of hosts.

4.1.2.1.2.2 Morphology

- They lack a digestive tract.
- They lack a defined circulatory system.
- Their tegument is a "naked" protoplasmic surface through which substances enter and leave.
- Nutritional.
- It is assumed that they utilize small molecules derived from host food sources.
- However, they can fix carbon dioxide (source of carbon atoms).
- They are known to utilize larger molecules by direct uptake.
- The scolex, e.g., in *Echinococcus*, is believed to have a placenta-like function in addition to its role of attachment.
- Carbohydrate metabolism is pronounced in cestodes.
- Most species utilize glucose, e.g., *H. diminuta/Taenia*, etc.
- Uptake of glucose is by active transport (operates against a concentration).
- They can also utilize galactose, which can also be absorbed by active transport.
- The E–M Pathology is operational in cestodes.
- Several enzymes for carbohydrates have been identified.
- Protein digestion occurs in cestodes; both large and small molecules of amino acids are absorbed.
- Amino-acid uptake is by active transport; however, the amino acid requirements are not known.
- Cestodes derive their fatty acid requirements entirely from their host. They cannot synthesize it de novo.
- Cestodes utilize a lot of cholesterol but are unable to synthesize it de novo.

4.1.3 PHYLUM NEMATODA (ROUNDWORMS)

- Body cavity or pseudocoelom is filled with pseudocoelomic/peri-enteric fluid or haemolymph.
- Haemolymph contains proteins/carbohydrates/fats and Hb.
- The main carbohydrate in nematodes is **glycogen**.
- The main proteins are **keratin/sclerotic** and **collagen**.
- Metabolism is anaerobic in nematodes, and some undergo complete Glycolysis.
- **Glycogen** is the main energy reserve/source.
- Unlike the adults, oxygen is required for the initiation and maintenance of eggs.
- Larval stages are obligate aerobes.

- Different larval stages may have different metabolic patterns, e.g., L3 – anaerobic with inactive Krebs cycle L2 – aerobic with active Krebs cycle L4 – anaerobic.
- Filaria worms have low glycogen concentration.
- Filaria worms undergo glycolytic metabolism.
- Amino acid is the chief source in filarial worms; however, in some species, glucose is the main energy source.
- Protein metabolism is not clear, although many proteolytic enzymes are known to be present.
- Amino acids do not act as an important source of energy.
- Nematodes that live under anaerobic conditions are not normally able to utilize lipids.
- Under aerobic conditions, however, lipids may be utilized for energy production.
- Carbohydrates/proteins/fats form the main nutritional requirements of adult worms.
- Several digestive enzymes are present and active in nematodes.

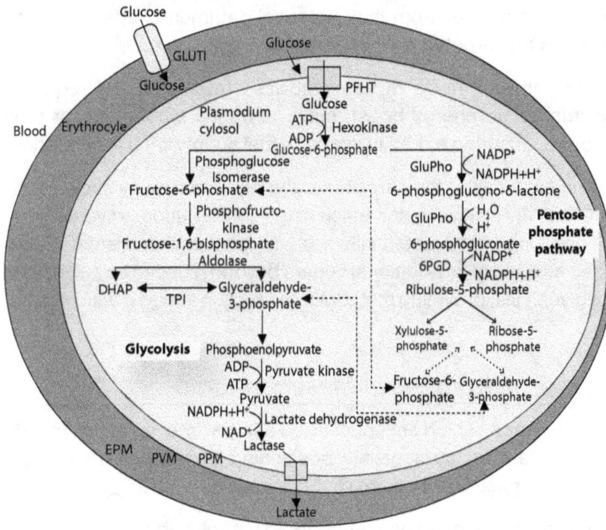

Figure 4.1 Glucose metabolism in *Plasmodium*-infected erythrocytes. Glucose enters the infected red blood cell via the host GLUT1 transporter. Once inside the erythrocyte cytosol, glucose is metabolized through two main pathways: Glycolysis and the pentose phosphate pathway (PPP).

4.2 METABOLIC PATHWAYS IN PARASITES

4.2.1 GLYCOLYSIS

Glycolysis is a metabolic pathway that converts glucose into pyruvate, occurring in the cytosol of both prokaryotic and eukaryotic cells. It is the first step in the breakdown of glucose to extract energy for cellular metabolism.

4.2.1.1 Glycolysis in Sarcodines

Sarcodine glycolysis unfolds within dedicated, mobile compartments known as **glycosomes**. The enzymes responsible for glucose breakdown reside not in a central location, but in these glycosomes. The glycosomes concentrate and isolate the glycolytic machinery, strategically positioning themselves near regions of high energy demand, such as the tips of extending pseudopods. This compartmentalized approach offers significant advantages for sarcodines. Potentially hazardous intermediates of the glycolytic process are encapsulated within the glycosomes, shielding the rest of the cell from their potential detrimental effects. It also enables the targeted distribution of energy resources.

Glycosomes can be rapidly mobilized towards areas requiring an immediate energy boost, such as during locomotion or prey capture, ensuring a readily available fuel supply wherever needed.

Some enzymes of the **sarcodine glycolytic pathway** show modified activity, allowing for efficient glycolysis under diverse conditions, including potentially low oxygen environments. Some species can utilize additional sugars beyond glucose as substrates for glycolysis, providing metabolic flexibility in varied environments.

4.2.1.2 Glycolysis in Mastigophorans

Glycosomes, which are specialized compartments, act as mobile power stations, strategically positioning themselves near high-demand areas like the base of the flagellum.

The mobile glycosomes can be rapidly deployed to areas requiring an immediate energy boost, ensuring a readily available fuel supply for flagellar motion, cell division, or even nutrient acquisition. They also act as metabolic shields, protecting the cell from the potentially toxic by-products of glycolysis.

4.2.1.3 Glycolysis in Apicomplexans

4.2.1.3.1 GLYCOLYSIS IN THE MALARIA PARASITE

In parasites, glycolysis plays a crucial role in their survival and proliferation. For instance, in the malaria parasite *Plasmodium falciparum*, glycolysis is the main pathway for ATP production and is essential for its survival.

Unlike conventional, cytoplasmic systems, Apicomplexan glycolysis occurs within membrane-bound compartments called **apicoplasts**.

Key intermediates, potentially toxic in the cytosol, are safely sequestered within the apicoplast boundaries. Additionally, some enzymes exhibit altered functionality, contributing to metabolic quirks unique to Apicomplexa.

Apoplasts, with their concentrated enzymatic repertoire, provide localized energy production near areas of high demand, like developing merozoites or invading host cell membranes. Furthermore, the sequestered intermediates and adapted enzymes shield both the parasite and the host cell from potential damage. This intricate metabolic machinery also contributes to crucial processes beyond glycolysis, including fatty acid synthesis, underscoring its vital role in parasite survival and virulence.

4.2.1.4 Glycolysis in Ciliates

Ciliates have organelles called **cytostomes** in which glycolysis occurs. Their glycolytic pathway changes depending on oxygen availability in the host. Some ciliates can switch between aerobic and anaerobic glycolysis.

Ciliates exhibit a wider range of end products compared to other phyla. While some produce lactate and/or ethanol, others may form acetate, propionate, or even hydrogen gas.

4.2.1.5 Glycolysis In Helminths

Glycolysis occurs in glycosomes in helminths. The presence of glycosomes introduces unique regulatory mechanisms, allowing the parasite to fine-tune energy production according to its specific needs and host environment. Glycolysis in helminths has an additional step, the conversion of pyruvate to lactate through anaerobic fermentation.

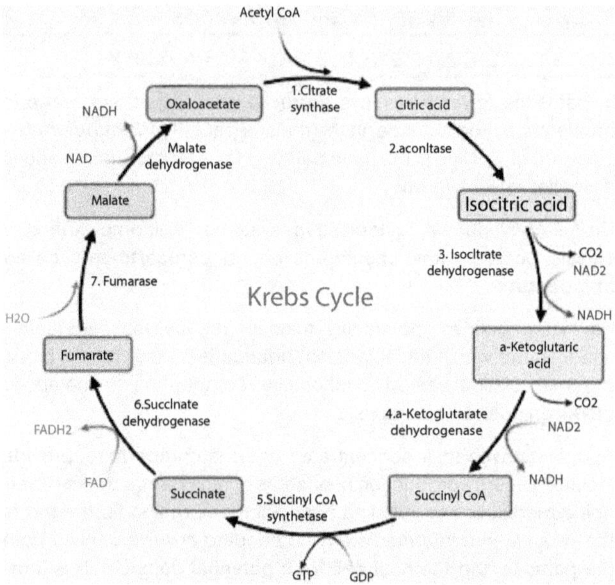

Figure 4.2 The tricarboxylic acid (TCA) cycle (Krebs cycle/ citric acid cycle). Acetyl CoA enters the cycle by condensing with oxaloacetate via citrate synthase (1) to form citric acid. A series of enzymatic reactions – catalysed by aconitase (2), isocitrate dehydrogenase (3), α-ketoglutarate dehydrogenase (4), succinyl CoA synthetase (5), succinate dehydrogenase (6), fumarase (7), and malate dehydrogenase (8–9) – lead to the regeneration of oxaloacetate (10). The cycle produces NADH, $FADH_2$, and CO_2 as byproducts, which drive oxidative phosphorylation and ATP synthesis.

Helminths can utilize alternative carbon sources beyond glucose, such as lipids or amino acids, demonstrating their ability to adjust their metabolism based on the available resources within their host.

4.2.1.6 Glycolysis In Ectoparasites

The glycolytic pathway of ectoparasites such as ticks is tuned for resilience, allowing them to conserve energy and survive on minimal glucose sources, such as host skin debris. This is because they face extended periods of starvation between meals. Other ectoparasites that do not utilize the glycolytic cycle rely on anaerobic fermentation.

4.2.2 KREBS CYCLE

The role of the Krebs cycle among parasites varies considerably. Reliance on the Krebs cycle is limited or even absent in some parasites. The Krebs cycle serves to oxidize acetyl-CoA, derived from carbohydrates or fatty acids, to generate ATP. Through a series of eight enzymatic steps, citrate undergoes various transformations, releasing energy in the form of ATP, NADH, and $FADH_2$. These energy carriers then feed into the electron transport chain, where they ultimately generate even more ATP.

The tricarboxylic acid cycle also plays several additional roles in the cell, including providing precursors for amino acid synthesis, regulating cellular redox balance and contributing to gluconeogenesis (glucose synthesis).

4.2.2.1 Krebs Cycle in Protozoa

Unlike their free-living counterparts which predominantly rely on glucose, parasitic protozoa exhibit remarkable flexibility in their choice of fuel sources. This metabolic agility allows them to thrive in diverse host niches despite limited access to their preferred sugars. Protozoans such as trypanosomes, *Leishmania* spp., and *Trichomonas* spp. use various sources such as fatty acids, complex sugars, amino acids, and lactate.

Modifications in Krebs cycle enzymes of parasites allow for efficient energy production. Variations in the parasite enzyme succinate dehydrogenase, and modifications to key regulatory enzymes make these enzymes less susceptible to host immune responses. Also, scattering of enzymes outside of the mitochondria in some parasites helps optimize metabolic transport and energy production.

4.2.2.2 Krebs Cycle in Helminths

Certain helminths, like tapeworms (phylum Platyhelminthes), lack mitochondria entirely and depend on alternative metabolic pathways such as anaerobic fermentation for energy. Many helminths live in environments with fluctuating oxygen levels. This necessitates metabolic flexibility, often shifting between aerobic and anaerobic pathways. Depending on their location and diet within the host, helminths may prioritize different energy sources. Some focus on metabolizing lipids while others primarily utilize carbohydrates. Some helminths harbour bacteria within their cells. These bacteria can contribute to the parasite's metabolism through additional pathways, potentially interacting with the Krebs cycle in complex ways.

4.2.3 THE ELECTRON TRANSPORT CHAIN

4.2.3.1 Electron Transport Chain in Protozoa

In aerobic environments, most protozoa follow the conventional mitochondrial ETC, utilizing oxygen as the terminal electron acceptor to generate ATP through oxidative phosphorylation. However, their parasitic lifestyle demands adaptability. Some parasites can switch between aerobic and anaerobic respiration.

Some species of parasites rely on alternative sources such as fumarate or nitrate in order to generate ATP through anaerobic pathways. Many species lack complex I, the first enzyme in the mitochondrial ETC, relying instead on alternative NADH dehydrogenase enzymes to feed electrons into the system.

Furthermore, some protozoa harbour endosymbiotic bacteria within their cells, and these bacteria often contribute to the parasite's overall ATP production through their own distinct ETCs. The combined activity of host and symbiont ETCs creates a complex metabolic network that optimizes energy production in these intricate parasitic relationships.

4.2.3.2 Electron Transport Chain in Helminths

The ETCs of helminths are predominantly geared towards anaerobic ATP production. The accumulation of reducing equivalents like NADH during glycolysis can disrupt cellular processes. To circumvent this, helminths employ alternative electron acceptors like fumarate or nitrate. NADH, regenerating NAD+ and preventing redox imbalance, reduces these acceptors. Additionally, some helminths, like *Ascaris lumbricoides*, utilize trans-sulphur metabolism as an alternative electron sink, further diversifying their anaerobic ATP production strategies.

4.3 DEFINITIONS

Cytostome: A mouth-like opening in certain protozoa used for ingesting food particles.

Micropore: A small channel-like opening in the tegument of cestodes (tapeworms) involved in nutrient absorption.

Plerocercoid: The infective larval stage of certain cestodes (e.g., Diphyllobothrium), found in the tissues of a second intermediate host, typically fish.

Paracostal: Referring to granules or fibers located alongside the costa (a rod-like structure) in certain flagellate protozoa such as Trichomonas.

Paraxostylar: Referring to granules or structures situated alongside the axostyle in flagellate protozoa.

Placental digestion: The process by which certain parasites, particularly Toxoplasma gondii and some helminths, break down and utilize placental tissue as a nutrient source, often facilitating transplacental transmission to the fetus.

FURTHER READING

Acosta-Virgen, K., Chávez-Munguía, B., Talamás-Lara, D., Lagunes-Guillén, A., Martínez-Higuera, A., Lazcano, A., Martínez-Palomo, A., & Espinosa-Cantellano, M. (2018). Giardia lamblia: Identification of peroxisomal-like proteins. *Experimental Parasitology*, 191, 36–43. https://doi.org/10.1016/J.EXPPARA.2018.06.006

Bártulos, C. R., Rogers, M. B., Williams, T. A., Gentekaki, E., Brinkmann, H., Cerff, R., Liaud, M. F., Hehl, A. B., Yarlett, N. R., Gruber, A., Kroth, P. G., & van der Giezen, M. (2018a). Mitochondrial glycolysis in a major lineage of eukaryotes. *Genome Biology and Evolution*, 10(9), 2310–2325. https://doi.org/10.1093/GBE/EVY164

Goerdeler, F., Seeberger, P. H., & Moscovitz, O. (2021a). Unveiling the sugary secrets of plasmodium parasites. *Frontiers in Microbiology*, 12, 712538. https://doi.org/10.3389/FMICB.2021.712538/BIBTEX

Kovářová, J., & Barrett, M. P. (2016). The pentose phosphate pathway in parasitic trypanosomatids. *Trends in Parasitology*, 32(8), 622–634. https://doi.org/10.1016/J.PT.2016.04.010

Krishnan, A., & Soldati-Favre, D. (2021). Amino acid metabolism in apicomplexan parasites. *Metabolites*, 11(2), 1–17. https://doi.org/10.3390/METABO11020061

Krüger, T., Schuster, S., & Engstler, M. (2018). Beyond blood: African trypanosomes on the move. *Trends in Parasitology*, 34(12), 1056–1067.

Moreira, R. S., Calomeno, N. A., das Neves, G. B., do Nascimento, L. F. N., Filho, V. B., Wagner, G., & Miletti, L. C. (2023). Trypanosoma evansi secretome carries potential biomarkers for Surra diagnosis. *Journal of Proteomics*, 272, 104789. https://doi.org/10.1016/j.jprot.2022.104789

Patra, J., Rana, D., Arora, S., Pal, M., & Mahindroo, N. (2023). Falcipains: Biochemistry, target validation and structure-activity relationship studies of inhibitors as antimalarials. In *European Journal of Medicinal Chemistry,* 252, 115299. https://doi.org/10.1016/j.ejmech.2023.115299

Roditi, I. (2016). The languages of parasite communication. *Molecular and Biochemical Parasitology*, 208(1), 16–22. https://doi.org/10.1016/j.molbiopara.2016.05.008

Saz, H. J. (1981). Energy metabolisms of parasitic helminths: adaptations to parasitism. *Annual Review of Physiology*, 43, 323–341. https://doi.org/10.1146/ANNUREV.PH.43.030181.00154

Shunmugam, S., Arnold, C. S., Dass, S., Nicholas, J. K., & Botté, C. Y. (2022). The flexibility of Apicomplexa parasites in lipid metabolism. *PLoS Pathogens*, 18(3), e1010313. https://doi.org/10.1371/JOURNAL.PPAT.1010313

Smithson, D. C., Lee, J., Shelat, A. A., Phillips, M. A., & Guy, R. K. (2010). Discovery of potent and selective inhibitors of Trypanosoma brucei ornithine decarboxylase. *Journal of Biological Chemistry*, 285(22), 16771–16781. https://doi.org/10.1074/jbc.M109.081588

Świderski, Z. & Georgiev, B. (2008). Fundamentals of Cestodology. Volume 14. Aploparaksidae of wild and domesticated birds, by S. K. Bondarenko and V. L. Kontrimavichus (Ed. S. O. Movsesyan). Published by NAUKA, Moscow, 2006. *Acta Parasitologica*, 53(1), 115–116. https://doi.org/10.2478/s11686-008-0014-y?

Timofeev, S., Tokarev, Y., & Dolgikh, V. (2020). Energy metabolism and its evolution in Microsporidia and allied taxa. *Parasitology Research*, 119(5), 1433–1441. https://doi.org/10.1007/S00436-020-06657-9/METRIC

Wangchuk, P., Yeshi, K., & Loukas, A. (2023a). Metabolomics and lipidomics studies of parasitic helminths: Molecular diversity and identification levels achieved by using different characterization tools. *Metabolomics*, 19(7), 1–23. https://doi.org/10.1007/S11306-023-02019-5/FIGURES/3

5 Epidemiology of Parasitic Infections

Action without thought is empty. Thought without action is blind.

Kwame Nkrumah

CHAPTER OUTLINE

In this chapter, we explore the fascinating world of epidemiology as it relates to parasitic infections. Here's what you can expect to learn:

- *Application of Parasite Epidemiology*: Identification of parasitic diseases in communities, detection of new/emerging parasitic infections, surveillance and outbreak prevention, investigation, and control of disease outbreaks, planning interventions and evaluating health programmes and describing the health status of human populations.
- *Concept of Disease Causation*: Understanding the roles of infectious agents, the environment, and hosts in disease occurrence, the interplay between these factors determines disease development and spread.
- *Transmission Modes and Factors*: Direct contact, vehicle, vector, and airborne transmission, environmental and host factors influencing transmission dynamics.
- *Environmental and Host Factors*: Exploring the impact of physical, biological, and social environments, understanding how host immunity and behaviours affect disease occurrence.
- *Levels of Parasitic Disease Prevention*: Primary, secondary, and tertiary prevention strategies; the importance of health promotion, exposure prevention, and disease prevention.
- *Epidemiologic Methods*: Observational and experimental approaches to studying disease dynamics, various study types, including cross-sectional, randomized controlled trials, and community trials.
- *Investigation of Parasitic Disease Outbreaks*: Identifying causes, modes of transmission, and environmental factors; the essential steps in investigating and managing outbreaks.

DOI: 10.1201/9781003733935-5

- *Global Prevalence and Distribution*: Examining the prevalence and impact of parasitic infections worldwide, understanding the burden of diseases such as malaria, schistosomiasis, strongyloidiasis, and others.

5.1 EPIDEMIOLOGY

Epidemiology is a descriptive science that involves the analysis of the determinants. Epidemiology of disease and other health-related conditions in a defined human population particularly describes disease occurrence, its distribution, and the impact on populations. Understanding the epidemiology of parasitic infections helps to identify risk factors and exposures, as well as helping to design strategies to prevent diseases.

Epidemiology is a crucial aspect of public health, which encompasses several other disciplines, including biology (to understand disease mechanisms), social sciences (to evaluate the dynamics of human behaviour in relation to disease), statistics (to generate data, make inferences through analysis and draw conclusions), and engineering (to design systems and infrastructure to limit disease causation and spread).

5.1.1 APPLICATION OF PARASITE EPIDEMIOLOGY

- To identify parasitic diseases plaguing communities.
- To detect new/emerging parasitic infections.
- For surveillance of parasitic diseases, to avert outbreaks.
- To investigate disease outbreaks.
- To plan interventions and strategies for parasitic disease control.
- To evaluate the efficacy of health programmes and interventions.
- To describe the health status of human populations.

5.1.2 CONCEPT OF DISEASE CAUSATION

There are three (3) major links in the causation of parasitic diseases:

- The infectious agent
- The environment
- The host

The concept of disease occurrence is multifactorial; however, the interaction among these three key factors (infectious agent, environment, and host) determines whether disease will develop, and the extent to which it can spread in populations. In most cases, an altered equilibrium within these interactive domains results in disease.

5.1.3 THE TREE

The schematic tree depicts the relationship between the factors responsible for the occurrence of parasitic diseases. Each factor plays an important role in the epidemiology of disease.

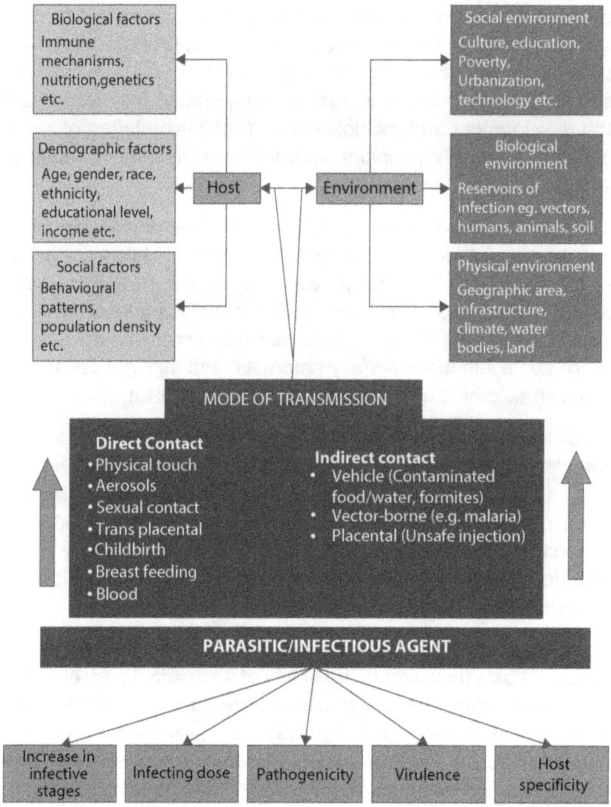

Figure 5.1 Conceptual framework showing interactions between host environment and parasitic/infectious agent, with direct and indirect transmission routes.

THE ROOT, which represents the parasitic/infectious agent, may be described as the primary cause of any parasitic disease. One of the reasons for disease occurrence is attributed to increased numbers of infective stages.

Infective stages of parasites may multiply seasonally depending on several factors such as climatic conditions, which often provide developmental stimuli. Availability of hosts (intermediate and definitive), host factors (temperature, CO_2, O_2, bile, nutrients, circadian rhythm), and parasite fecundity may all result in the multiplication of infective stages.

Some species of Ascaris produce many thousands of eggs daily due to their fecundity, while other parasites like *Trichostrongylus* produce only a few hundred. Ectoparasites such as the blowfly, *Lucilia sericata*, or the tick, *Ixodes ricinus*, also produce high numbers of eggs, whereas *Glossina* spp. produce relatively few offspring. Climatic conditions such as temperature may also affect the development and multiplication of infective stages of some parasites, e.g., *Plasmodium* sporozoites within the Anopheles vector.

The infecting dose of the parasitic agent determines whether or not disease will develop. Usually, host immune defence mechanisms can stave off most parasitic infections. Properties such as pathogenicity and virulence of the infectious agent, however, could intensify the morbidity of parasitic diseases on populations. While some infections are asymptomatic and may not cause disease, some others could be pathogenic and virulent.

Parasites such as *Echinococcus granulosus*, *Trypanosoma* spp., *Naegleria fowleri*, and *Taenia solium* are considered highly virulent and invasive due to their ability to cross the blood–brain barrier. Such properties may influence disease severity and morbidity. Compared to others, the extent of damage produced by these infections may be more pronounced in populations, particularly when infective stages are multiplied.

Again, most parasites are host specific, while some others have a range of hosts they infect. The ability of a parasite to infect different host species (humans and vertebrate animals) can affect the dynamics of epidemiology. Parasitic zoonoses such as trichinosis, cryptosporidiosis, toxoplasmosis, among others, are usually encountered when the barriers between humans and animals are broken, and the equilibrium within the environment is distorted. This may often result in disease outbreaks, posing a serious threat to populations.

THE TRUNK indicates the various modes of the transmission of parasitic agents to the host and the environment. This is probably the most important link in disease occurrence since it characterizes the various means by which the infectious agent moves from the source to the host, and how it is shed into the environment. The principal modes of parasite transmission are by direct contact, by a vehicle, through a vector, or through the air.

Direct contact transmission is seen in parasites such as *Schistosoma* spp. (through contact with waterbodies containing infective stages), *Trichomonas vaginalis* (through sexual contact with an infected person), hookworms, and *Strongyloides* spp. (via contact with faecally polluted soil), *Pediculus humanus* (via head-to-head contact), *Toxoplasma gondii* (transmission of tachyzoites through blood transfusion, breastfeeding, and from pregnant mother to child transplacentally, in the uterus or at birth).

Direct contact transmission facilitates the life cycle of parasites and propagates infective stages such that over time, a stock of infectious microorganisms remains within the environment. A high stock density of parasites within the environment eventually produces reservoirs of infection that favour spread among populations and consequently reinforce the disease cycle.

Parasites can also be transmitted through inanimate objects such as food, water, and drugs. Drinking from contaminated water sources, eating fruits and vegetables without washing, or eating raw/undercooked meat or fish renders these objects vehicles of transmission to propagate parasitic infections among communities.

Entamoeba histolytica, *Giardia lamblia*, *Enterobius vermicularis*, *Dracunculus medinensis*, *Echinococcus granulosus*, *Hymenolepis nana*, *Taenia solium*, *Fasciola hepatica*, *and Paragonimus westermani* are all examples of parasites transmitted through vehicles.

Some parasites are also transmitted through biological vectors like arthropods. *Babesia* spp. is transmitted by the tick, *Ixodes scapularis*; *Plasmodium* spp. by Anopheles mosquito; *Leishmania* spp. by Phlebotomus sandfly; *Loa loa* by horseflies*; Onchocerca volvulus* by the Simulium blackfly, and filarial worms by mosquitoes. Vector bionomics, human behaviour, and environmental factors play unique roles in the exposures and outcomes of these vector-borne parasitic infections.

Few parasites are transmitted through the air. Hydatid cysts of *Echinococcus granulosus* may be transmitted directly into the respiratory tract from eggs blown in dust by wind. Rarely, *Cryptosporidium* oocysts may also be transmitted through inhalation of aerosolized droplets. Exposures are particularly dependent on environmental factors and the stock density of infective stages.

THE BRANCHES of the schematic tree are represented by host and environmental factors. Host and environmental factors are interconnected and interactive, and as such, deviations from this congruous intercourse usually influence the health equilibrium.

5.2 THE ENVIRONMENT

The environment comprises all external factors that contribute to parasitic disease occurrence. These factors may be categorized as physical, biological, or social. The physical environment takes into consideration natural and artificial resources, climate, infrastructure, etc. and how this affects epidemiology.

Water bodies and land fields may serve as reservoirs from which many parasitic diseases could be transmitted. Climatic factors have also been shown to influence the infective stages of many parasites and the prevalence of some intermediate hosts. For example, temperature could assist or inhibit the multiplication of parasites at their reservoir. A high prevalence of *Fasciola hepatica* in ruminants has been associated with warmer, wetter seasons.

High rainfall patterns lead to the proliferation of mosquito breeding habitats, thereby increasing the potential for vector-borne diseases like malaria. Air velocity could also assist the airborne movement of droplet nuclei to propagate infection. Furthermore, low humidity has been shown to damage mucous membranes to facilitate parasite entry into hosts.

The biological environment mainly consists of the soil, plants, animals, humans, vectors, etc., which could potentially serve as reservoirs of infection. Soil conditions and herbage may favour the development and survival of helminth larvae, ticks, larval stages of insects, and coccidia oocysts. While different vertebrate animals may act as intermediate/definite hosts of many parasitic infections, some invertebrate vectors could also harbour and develop many parasites for transmission.

Human invasion into previously unoccupied areas results in interactions with domestic and wild animal reservoirs, which often leads to the outbreak of zoonotic diseases. The emergence and persistence of zoonosis in human populations may over time lead to the evolution of novel variants, making it difficult to break the infection cycle. Human behavioural patterns and food habits may also result in gene mixes with parasite-infected animals, thereby fuelling transmission.

The One Health concept therefore considers health in the context of human, animal, and the environment. It addresses health crises arising from the human–animal–ecosystem interface with approaches directed at preventing zoonotic disease outbreaks and protecting biodiversity.

The social environment consists of elements pertaining to culture, economy, education, technology, and politics, to mention a few. Certain cultural norms and practices may influence the dynamics of disease transmission negatively. For instance, eating raw meat/fish as it is in some cultures, walking barefoot, exposing dead humans to dogs and hyenas, gender roles, reliance on traditional healers, belief in myths, etc. allow the dissemination of many parasite species.

Poverty is associated with other social challenges such as lack of basic amenities, malnutrition, poor sanitation, low levels of education, inadequate public health infrastructure, among other factors, which ultimately facilitate the propagation of parasitic infections.

5.3 THE HOST

The occurrence of a parasitic disease within the host is influenced by biological factors such as immune barriers and mechanisms including the skin, mucous membranes, secretions, excretions, enzymes, inflammatory response, specific antibodies, immune cells, as well as nutrition and genetics.

Host immunity limits the level of contamination in the environment by modifying the development of new infections either by their destruction or arrest at the larval stages, while existing adult worm burdens are either expelled or their egg production severely curtailed. Conversely, low/absence of host immunity facilitates the spread of infections.

In protozoal diseases such as babesiosis, the presence of immune adults limits the likelihood of ticks becoming infected, thus truncating the infection cycle. On the other hand, resistance to intestinal protozoal infections such as coccidiosis and toxoplasmosis has been shown to be lowered during pregnancy and lactation, thereby enhancing spread.

Social factors such as certain human behavioural patterns may promote the dissemination of parasitic infections within populations; poor sanitation, poor hygiene, sexual promiscuity, and some cultural practices have been demonstrated to enhance the spread of protozoal infections such as *Entamoeba histolytica*, *Giardia lamblia*, *Trichomonas vaginalis*, *Toxoplasma gondii*, as well as nematodes (*Trichuris trichiura*, hookworms, roundworms, tapeworms) and trematodes (*Fasciola hepatica*, *Schistosoma* spp.).

Demographic factors such as age, race, gender, and ethnicity, among others, may predispose certain populations to parasitic infections. Low immunity is mostly associated with children under 5 years old, and as such, a high prevalence of certain parasitic diseases may be recorded in this group, e.g., malaria.

Some parasitic infections have also been associated more with certain ethnic groups or races, and they keep spreading among such populations because of geographic, socioeconomic, and sociocultural factors peculiar to these groups. Africa, for instance, accounts for a high proportion of global parasitic diseases. A classic example is the neglected tropical diseases (NTDs) burden.

Ascariasis, dracunculiasis, hookworm infections, African trypanosomiasis, leishmaniasis, lymphatic filariasis, onchocerciasis, trichuriasis and schistosomiasis are all examples of NTDs plaguing the region. Several other factors may influence the occurrence of parasitic diseases. The interconnections among the key factors discussed in this section, however, greatly influence the dynamics of epidemiology.

5.4 LEVELS OF PARASITIC DISEASE PREVENTION

5.4.1 *PRIMARY PREVENTION*

It is foremost, and it aims at promoting health, preventing exposures, and diseases. Thus, interventions that enhance health, such as regular exercise, recreation, good nutrition, good housing, health education, good working conditions, healthcare infrastructure, etc., all constitute health promotion. Exposure prevention, on the other hand, deals with refraining from exposure factors that cause disease, whereas disease prevention involves methods such as vaccination.

5.4.2 SECONDARY PREVENTION

Limits the progression of disease or prevents complications, in order to avert permanent damage. It is achieved through early diagnosis and prompt treatment of individuals who have a particular disease.

5.4.3 TERTIARY PREVENTION

It is aimed at preventing further disability or death. It deals with limiting the physical, psychological, social, and financial impact of disability, so as to improve the quality of life. Rehabilitation is an example of tertiary prevention.

5.5 EPIDEMIOLOGIC METHODS

Epidemiologic studies provide varied approaches to obtaining epidemiological data. The methods may either be observational or experimental.

Observational epidemiology bifurcates into descriptive epidemiology (which describes the frequency and distribution of diseases and other health-related conditions by time, place, and person) and analytical epidemiology (which deals with the causes or determinants of diseases), e.g., cross-sectional studies or surveys

Experimental epidemiology uses an organized approach to problem solving. It involves three case types: Randomized controlled trials (often used for a new medicine or drug testing), field trials (conducted on those at a high risk of contracting a disease), and community trials (research on socially originating diseases).

5.5.1 SOURCES OF EPIDEMIOLOGICAL DATA

Information obtained from these sources is valuable in determining the health status of populations, investigating disease outbreaks, planning interventions, and evaluating health programmes. Some sources of epidemiological data have been listed.

- Health service records
- Health surveys: Surveys of specific parasitic diseases, e.g., lymphatic filariasis, schistosomiasis, hookworm infections, etc.

- Census
- Vital statistics, e.g., registration of births and deaths

5.5.2 MEASUREMENTS OF HEALTH

These are parameters used to measure health and disease outcomes in relation to a population at risk.

Incidence measures the frequency of disease. It refers to the number of new cases reported over a specified period in a defined population.

Prevalence also measures the frequency of disease. It refers to the number of people who have a particular disease at a point in time (point prevalence) or over a period (period prevalence). Period prevalence gives a clearer picture because it includes all individuals with old and new (incident) cases, as well as those who were cured or died during the period.

Rates express the frequency of a characteristic per 1,000 (10,000 or 100,000) persons in the population. Rates are used to compare the frequency of disease in different groups. A rate is calculated by dividing the numerator (e.g., number of cases) by the denominator (the population at risk).

Prevalence rate: The numerator in this case is the prevalence, and the denominator is the population at risk. For example: If there are six individuals with *Ascaris lumbricoides* infection at a specified time within a population size of 100, then the prevalence rate = reported as; 60 per 1,000 (or 600 per 10,000 or 6,000 per 100,000).

Incidence rate and cumulative incidence: The incidence rate takes into account the length of time each individual in the population at risk was under observation until disease onset or loss to follow-up, in terms of person-time (person-days, person-months, or person-years). On the other hand, the cumulative incidence assumes that the entire population at risk is followed up for the specified period.

Incidence rate =

Reported as the number of cases per unit time.

Cumulative incidence =

Entire at risk population followed over a period of time.

Crude and specific rates: The total number of cases in a population at risk is generally regarded as a crude or overall rate.

However, it is more interesting to know the rates for subgroups within the population, for example, for the sexes or for different age groups. These are referred to as specific rates.

Mortality rate: The mortality rate is the ratio of the number of deaths due to a disease to the average total population in a year.

Case fatality: The proportion of people who die from a specified disease among all individuals diagnosed with the disease over a certain period. Case fatality rate typically is used as a measure of disease severity and is often used for prognosis.

Disability adjusted life years (DALYs): The sum of the years of life lost due to premature mortality and the years lived with a disability due to prevalent cases of the disease or health condition in a population.

5.6 INVESTIGATION OF PARASITIC DISEASE OUTBREAKS

A parasitic disease outbreak is the sudden rise in the incidence of a specific parasitic disease within a vulnerable population. The cases usually occur in excess and cover a more limited area. Generally, the cause of an outbreak is mostly unknown until an investigation is carried out.

Most parasitic disease outbreaks are influenced by environmental factors such as water supply, sanitation, food, air quality, and climate. Lack of potable water, unsafe/contaminated food, poor hygiene practices, inadequate excreta disposal facilities, and poor living conditions can all cause parasitic diarrhoeal diseases that could potentially spread among affected populations within the shortest possible time.

Climate can influence outbreaks by diverse means. For instance, flooding after heavy rains can cause sewage overflow and widespread water contamination. Stagnant water that remains after heavy rains can also serve as breeding sites/reservoirs for parasitic vectors/infective stages. It has also been shown that pathogens can be spread from one region to another along air streams or by wind, e.g., hydatid cysts of *Echinococcus granulosus*.

Investigating a parasitic disease outbreak is essential in controlling it and avoiding future occurrences. The approach involves asking vital questions.

i. Which infectious agent is responsible for the outbreak?
ii. What is the principal mode of transmission?

iii. What specific sources can be identified?
iv. What environmental factors or behavioural patterns have contributed to the outbreak?
v. What chain of events led to the outbreak?

The investigation steps involve:

I. Data collection, e.g., number of disease cases, hospitalizations, deaths resulting from cases.
II. Clinical/laboratory diagnosis of reported cases.
III. Setting criteria to differentiate cases from non-cases.
IV. Describing the outbreak with respect to person, place and time using standard epidemiological parameters.
V. Identifying the cause of the outbreak.
VI. Management of the outbreak and follow-up actions.
VII. Reporting the investigation.

5.7 GLOBAL PREVALENCE AND DISTRIBUTION OF PARASITIC INFECTIONS

Intestinal parasitic infections, including Ascariasis (1.2 billion cases), hookworm infection (700–900 million cases), amoebiasis (500 million cases), trichuriasis (795 million cases), and *Giardia lamblia* (200 million cases) are the most prevalent in the world, carrying a high burden of morbidity and mortality, especially in developing countries.

Epidemiological studies across the world have shown that demographic characteristics, environmental, and socioeconomic factors aggravate the incidence of intestinal parasitic infections. In Sub-Saharan African countries, up to 250 million people are estimated to be infected with at least one or more species of these parasites. Compared to the general population, children of 5–14 years are most affected, representing 12% of the global disease burdens caused by intestinal parasites.

Intestinal parasitic infections have been listed among the topmost outpatient morbidities in Ghana. Prevalence is between 2% and 78% for various parasites and specific population groups.

Malaria is a major public health issue with an estimated 247 million cases and 619,000 mortalities worldwide. Sub-Saharan Africa represents the majority of all cases (95%) and deaths (96%), with children under 5 years accounting for about 80% of all malaria deaths in the region. Distribution of malaria parasites *Plasmodium falciparum, P. vivax, P. ovale, and P. malariae* varies geographically; however, the most pathogenic species, *Plasmodium falciparum*, accounts for more than 90% of malaria mortality in Sub-Saharan Africa.

Schistosomiasis is mainly endemic in Sub-Saharan Africa, accounting for 93% of all global cases, with *S. mansoni* and *S. haematobium* being the most implicated species. Outside the continent, schistosomiasis is classified among the persistent parasitic diseases among migrants, with 11–44% prevalence.

Strongyloidiasis is endemic in tropical and subtropical regions of the world, particularly showing asymptomatic chronic intestinal infection in immunocompetent individuals. In immunocompromised persons, however, the parasite invades the gastrointestinal and pulmonary systems (hyperinfection syndrome) and other organs (disseminated strongyloidiasis), resulting in high mortality rates (up to 87%). It is also classified among the persistent parasitic diseases among migrants, with 7.5–42% prevalence.

Paragonimiasis is endemic throughout Asia and West Africa, and globally, it is estimated that 20 million people are affected. The commonest complication of the disease is meningoencephalitis, which may persist for weeks. The mortality rate is up to 5% if left untreated.

Naegleria fowleri infection is known to be present throughout the world, with fewer than 100 reported cases. Most infections occur especially in children who wade in stagnant freshwater. This fatal amoebic disease primarily affects the central nervous system, particularly the brain, and has a mortality rate of up to 95%.

Human African Trypanosomiasis affects populations in **Sub-Saharan Africa**. The infection is common among individuals who live in rural areas and are involved in agricultural activities, fishing, and hunting. Most infections are attributed to *Trypanosoma brucei gambiense* (92% of reported cases), which is prevalent in 24 countries of West and Central Africa, whereas *Trypanosoma brucei rhodesiense*, found in 13 countries of Eastern and Southern Africa, accounts for 8% of reported cases. Ghana has experienced sporadic cases in the last decade.

Leishmaniasis is globally considered part of the ten (10) neglected tropical diseases, accounting for more than 12 million cases worldwide. It poses a serious public health threat in the Americas, East Africa, North Africa, and Western and Southeast

Asia. While leishmaniasis is endemic in 99 countries, cutaneous and visceral leishmaniasis are endemic in 89 countries and 80 countries respectively. In 71 countries, however, the two clinical forms (CL and VL) are endemic. Visceral leishmaniasis has a high mortality rate of more than 90%.

Toxoplasmosis is known to affect one-third of the world's population. The prevalence of the disease (10–80%) varies by geographical location, with the highest burden observed in areas with hot, humid climates and lower altitudes. Low prevalence has been observed in North America, Southeast Asia, Northern Europe, and Sahelian countries of Africa. Moderate prevalence has been found in countries of Central and Southern Europe, and high prevalence has been found in Latin America and in tropical African countries. Transmission is through congenital means from mother to child, blood transfusion, and organ transplantation.

Filariasis affects over 882 million people in 44 countries worldwide. Three (3) different species of filarial worms (*Wuchereria bancrofti* [90% of cases], *Brugia malayi*, and *Brugia timori*) cause lymphatic filariasis in humans. Mosquitoes act as the vectors of these parasites; in Africa, the most common vector is Anopheles, in the Americas, it is *Culex quinquefasciatus*, and in the Pacific and Asia, *Aedes* and *Mansoni* spp. transmit the infection. Lymphatic filariasis is usually asymptomatic; however, chronic conditions lead to lymphedema, elephantiasis of limbs, and hydrocele.

5.8 GLOBAL BURDEN OF PARASITIC INFECTIONS

Parasitic infections have become a rather disturbing development in our current ecosystem. It has, in recent years, garnered some attention. The World Health Organization estimates that at least one in six people worldwide are thought to be infected with a parasitic disease. This statistic starkly puts into perspective the need to understand immunology and how parasitic infections and parasites in themselves impact the general immunology of living beings.

5.9 DEFINITIONS

Parasite fecundity *is defined as the reproductive capacity of a parasite, typically measured by the number of offspring (such as eggs) produced by a single parasite or parasite population.*

FURTHER READING

Awasthi, S., Bundy, D., & Savioli, L. (2003). Helminthic infections. *BMJ*, 323, 431–433.

Centers for Disease Control and Prevention. (2018). *Parasites – Toxoplasmosis*. Global Health, Division of Parasitic Diseases and Malaria.

Chelkeba L., Mekonnen, Z., Alemu, Y., & Emana, D. (2020). Epidemiology of intestinal parasitic infections in preschool and school-aged Ethiopian children: A systematic review and meta-analysis. *BMC Public Health,* 20(1), 117.

Blair, D., Xu, Z. B., & Agatsuma, T. (1999). Paragonimiasis and the genus Paragonimus. *Advances in Parasitology*, 42, 113–222.

Duedu, K., Peprah, E., Anim-Baidoo, I., & Ayeh-Kumi, P. F. (2015). Prevalence of intestinal parasites and association with malnutrition at a Ghanaian Orphanage. *Human Parasitic Diseases*, 5. https://doi.org/10.4137/HPD.S30059

Duedu, K., Karikari, Y. A., Attah, S. K., & Ayeh-Kumi, P. F. (2015). Prevalence of intestinal parasites among patients of a Ghanaian psychiatry hospital. *BMC Research Notes*, 8.

Hailu, T., Abera, B., Mulu, W., Kassa, S., Genanew, A., & Amor, A. (2020). Prevalence and factors associated with intestinal parasitic infections among pregnant women in West Gojjam Zone, Northwest Ethiopia. *Journal of Parasitology Research*, 2020, 8855362. https://doi.org/10.1155/2020/8855362

Hotez, P. J., & Kamath, A. (2009). Neglected tropical diseases in sub-Saharan Africa: Review of their prevalence, distribution, and disease burden. *PLoS Neglected Tropical Diseases*, 3(8), e412.

Hochberg, N. S., Moro, R. N., Sheth, A. N., et al. (2011). High prevalence of persistent parasitic infections in foreign-born, HIV-infected persons in the United States. *PLoS Neglected Tropical Diseases*, 5, 4.

Jain, R., Prabhakar, S., & Modi, M. (2023). *Naegleria meningitis: A rare survival. Neurol India. 2002 World Health Organization. Trypanosomiasis, human African (Sleeping sickness). A report.* WHO.

Marcos, L. A., Terashima, A., Canales, M., & Gotuzzo, E. (2011). Update on strongyloidiasis in the immunocompromised host. *Current Infectious Disease Reports*, 13(1), 35–46.

Pan African Health Organization and World Health Organization. (2023). *Leishmaniasis. A report.* PANHO, WHO.

Pappas, G., Roussos, N., & Falagas, M. E. (2009). Toxoplasmosis snapshots: Global status of Toxoplasma gondii seroprevalence and implications for pregnancy and congenital toxoplasmosis. *International Journal for Parasitology*, 39, 1385–1394.

Salvador, F., Molina, I., Sulleiro, E., et al. (2013). Tropical diseases screening in immigrant patients with human immunodeficiency virus infection in Spain. *The American Journal of Tropical Medicine and Hygiene*, 88(6), 1196–1202.

Snow, R. W. (2015). Global malaria eradication and the importance of Plasmodium falciparum epidemiology in Africa. *BMC Medicine*, 13(1), 14–16. https://doi.org/10.1186/s12916-014-0254-7

World Health Organization. (1987). *Prevention and control of intestinal parasitic infections: report of a WHO Expert Committee* [meeting held in Geneva from 3 to 7 March 1986]: World Health Organization.

World Health Organization. (2023). *Lymphatic filariasis. A report.* WHO.

6 Immunology of Parasites and Their Hosts

Education is not a way to escape poverty; it is a way of fighting it.

Julius Nyerere

CHAPTER OUTLINE

In this chapter, we delve into the fascinating world of parasite–host interactions through the lens of immunology. Here's what you can expect to explore:

- *Global Burden of Parasitic Infections*: Explore the significant impact of parasitic infections on global health and the urgency for understanding their immunology.
- *Host Immune System and Co-evolution with Parasites*: Delve into the intricate interplay between parasites and the host's immune system, shaping evolutionary adaptations.
- *Structure and Function of Innate and Adaptive Immune Systems*: Understand the roles of innate and adaptive immunity in combating parasitic infections.
- *Parasite Immune Evasion Strategies*: Explore the sophisticated mechanisms parasites employ to evade and manipulate host immune responses.
- *Types of Immune Responses*: Learn about humoral and cell-mediated immunity and their roles in combating parasites.
- *Immune Responses to Different Parasite Types*: Understand how the immune system responds differently to protozoa, helminths, and ectoparasites.
- *Immune Pathology and Regulation*: Explore how immune responses to parasites can sometimes lead to harmful effects and how the immune system regulates itself.
- *Co-evolution and Immunological Adaptations*: Delve into the ongoing molecular arms race between parasites and hosts, shaping their evolution.
- *Examples of Co-evolutionary Arms Races*: Learn about specific examples of co-evolution between parasites and hosts, such as malaria and humans.

DOI: 10.1201/9781003733935-6

- *Potential Impact of Co-evolution on Vaccine Development*: Understand the challenges and opportunities co-evolution presents for vaccine development.
- *Future Directions and Challenges*: Explore emerging research areas and the challenges in controlling parasitic diseases.

6.1 HOST IMMUNE SYSTEM AND CO-EVOLUTION BETWEEN PARASITES

Immunology as a science is a fast adapting and researched aspect of science, as we know it now. It involves the study of the immune system, which is a complex combination of organs, cells, and chemicals that protect the body from harmful bacteria, viruses, and other attackers that can pose a threat to a living being. It is made up of two types: Innate and adaptive.

Parasites constitute some of the threats that face the function of the immune system of living beings. However, parasites have developed multifaceted strategies to utilize, evade, modulate, and regulate the host immune response to avoid elimination and ensure long-term survival. These multifaceted strategies are often specific to the different stages of the parasite's life cycle. Some of these processes would be expatiated later. With the host exerting selective pressures on parasites, causing adaptations in parasites. This co-evolution is ubiquitous and of potential importance to all living organisms, including humans. Major diseases such as malaria, AIDS, and influenza are caused by co-evolving parasites. A deeper understanding into co-evolving parasites could be the basis to understanding and developing novel medications and vaccines against these diseases.

6.1.1 STRUCTURE AND FUNCTION OF THE INNATE AND ADAPTIVE IMMUNE SYSTEMS

6.1.1.1 Innate Immune System

The innate immune system, also known as non-specific immunity, is the defensive mechanism present at birth. Its basic function is to protect against all antigens. It comprises physical barriers such as the skin, the gastrointestinal tract lining and secretions (mucus or saliva) and a variety of cells that act quickly and non-specifically against elements that are foreign to the host. Once a foreign substance invades the host's physical barrier, cells belonging to the inflammatory response are called into effect. These could include phagocyte cells, inflammatory mediator releasing cells, and natural killer cells to fight any intruder. However, it is worth noting that the innate immune system does not recognize every possible antigen.

6.1.1.2 Adaptive Immune System

The adaptive immune system is a type of immunity built up as the host is exposed to diseases or is vaccinated. This system is also known as the acquired immune system. As the host is continually exposed to specific antigens, it builds specificity in attacking these antigens should they arise another time. The adaptive system is able to achieve this specificity with the aid of two kinds of white blood cells to target pathogens: Namely, B cells and T cells. These cells arise from the bone marrow and the thymus respectively.

Parasites, as earlier mentioned, have developed multifaceted strategies to utilize, evade, modulate, and regulate the host immune response to avoid elimination and ensure their long-term survival. Some key components involved in parasitic defence include:

Camouflage: Parasites can become camouflaged by host factors to avoid detection.

Immune privileged sites: Parasites can inhabit immune privileged sites. These are areas of the body that can tolerate the introduction of antigens without eliciting an inflammatory immune response.

Stage-specific antigens: Parasites can express stage-specific antigens, which means they produce different antigens at different stages of their life cycle.

TABLE 6.1 Comparison of Innate and Adaptive Immune Systems

Feature	*Innate Immune System*	*Adaptive Immune System*
Development	Present at birth	Develops over time
Specificity	Non-specific	Highly specific
Response time	Immediate	Slower
Memory	No memory	Memory cells for long-term immunity

Mimicry: Parasites can secrete components that mimic host factors, thereby deceiving the host's immune system.

Immune cell differentiation: Parasites can drive the differentiation of immune cell phenotypes, influencing the host's immune response.

Regulation of host immune cells: Parasites can regulate the responsiveness of host immune cells, controlling how they react to the presence of the parasite. It is worth noting that with all the above mentioned, there is still an incomplete understanding of this relationship, and future research will be informed by concomitant developments in immunological, molecular, and cell culturing techniques and innovations.

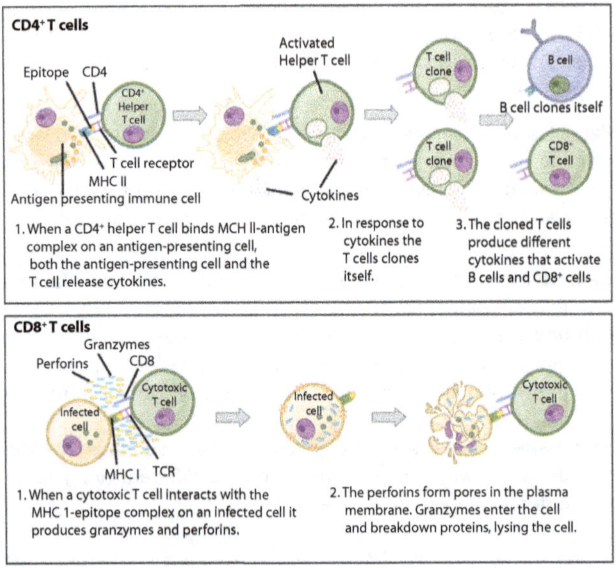

Figure 6.1 Clonal expansion of T cells following antigen recognition. Upon activation by infected cells, CD4+ helper T cells and CD8+ cytotoxic T cells undergo clonal proliferation, generating multiple clones of each cell type. The expanded CD4+ helper T cells assist other immune cells, while CD8+ cytotoxic T cells target and eliminate infected cells.

6.2 TYPES OF IMMUNE RESPONSE

1. ***Humoral immunity***: This immunity is mediated by B cells and antibodies. It is most effective against extracellular pathogens. The antibodies produced by the B cells bind to the antigens and neutralize the microbes. Humoral immunity shows a quick response against pathogens.
2. ***Cell-mediated immunity***: This type of immunity is facilitated by T-helper and cytotoxic T cells. It is most effective against intracellular pathogens. Cytokines secreted by the T-helper cells activate phagocytic cells, which phagocytose the pathogens and kill them. Cell-mediated immunity shows a delayed response.

Both humoral and cell-mediated immunity are active immunities, have a lag period, are active against a wide variety of pathogens, possess immunological memories, and are not effective in immune-deficient individuals.

6.2.1 PARASITE IMMUNE EVASION STRATEGIES

This section aims to explore the complex mechanisms employed by parasites to evade the host's immune system. These strategies, while detrimental to the host, provide fascinating insights into the evolving maze of survival and adaptation.

Parasites, as a part of their survival strategy, have evolved sophisticated mechanisms to evade the host's immune response. These mechanisms will shed light on the biological arms race between parasites and their hosts, and they include:

- Surface Antigen Variation
- Intracellular Parasitism
- Immune Decoy Release
- Immune Response Manipulation

6.2.2 PARASITE MECHANISMS TO AVOID IMMUNE DETECTION AND DESTRUCTION

Parasites have evolved a variety of strategies to evade the host's immune system. Here are some of the key mechanisms:

- ***Antigenic variation***: Parasites can alter their surface proteins to avoid recognition by the host's immune system. This antigenic variation allows parasites to persist in the host, leading to chronic infections. An example of a parasite that employs this mechanism is the African trypanosome, which causes sleeping sickness, frequently changes its surface proteins to avoid detection by the host's immune system.
- ***Immunosuppression***: Some parasites can suppress the host's immune response. They do this by releasing specific immunomodulatory factors that affect immune cell functions. This allows the parasites to establish and maintain an infection. An example is the *Leishmania* parasite, which causes Leishmaniasis and can selectively inhibit the transcription of the pro-inflammatory cytokine interleukin 12 (IL-12p40) in the host, thus suppressing the host's immune response.
- ***Camouflage (molecular mimicry)***: Parasites can mimic host antigens, effectively camouflaging themselves from the host's immune system. This allows them to travel undetected as they move between cells. An example is the Lyme disease-causing bacterium, *Borrelia burgdorferi*, which can mimic host antigens, effectively camouflaging itself from the host's immune system
- ***Intracellular parasitism***: Some parasites hide within the host's cells to evade immune detection. This strategy not only provides a safe haven for the parasites but also allows them to manipulate the host's cellular machinery for their benefit. Examples include viruses such as varicella zoster (chickenpox) and *Herpesviridae* (herpes simplex viruses, varicella zoster virus, cytomegalovirus, etc.) that can hide from the immune system in neurons and non-neuronal cells where they may persist for many years.
- ***Protease secretion***: Certain parasites secrete potent proteases, which can degrade the host's immune proteins, thereby disrupting the immune response. An example is the parasite that causes Chagas disease, *Trypanosoma cruzi*, which secretes proteases that can degrade the host's immune proteins, disrupting the immune response.
- ***Antibody trapping***: Some parasites have developed a mechanism to trap antibodies, preventing them from binding to the parasite's surface and marking it for destruction. An example is the schistosome parasite, which causes schistosomiasis and has been shown to trap antibodies, preventing them from binding to the parasite's surface and marking it for destruction.

Each of these mechanisms may be employed to varying degrees on the host by the parasite and generate in most cases, life-threatening implications, especially when they are not detected early enough for appropriate treatment to commence.

6.2.3 IMMUNE RESPONSES TO DIFFERENT PARASITE TYPES

Parasites encompass a wide range of organisms such as protozoa, helminths, and insects, and have evolved complex mechanisms to evade the host's immune system. As with all intrusions, the host employs its multifaceted immune defences specific to parasitic attacks, including both innate and adaptive immunity, and varies significantly depending on the type of parasite. Of these mechanisms, a few stand out and include:

- ***Intracellular protozoa***: Infections by intracellular protozoa typically elicit a TH1 immune response, involving macrophages (M1), interferon gamma (IFN?) CD4 T cells, innate lymphoid cells 1 (NKp44+ ILC1), CD8 T cells (Effector-Memory4, EM4), invariant natural killer T cells 1 (iNKT1) cells, and immunoglobulin G3 (IgG3) B cells. However, some intracellular protozoa can tolerate a TH1-like immune response, involving macrophages (M2), IFN?/TGF? CD4 T cells, NKp44- ILC1, CD8 T cells (EM3), iNKT1 cells, and IgA1 B cells.
- ***Extracellular protozoa***: Free-living extracellular protozoa typically elicit a TH22 immune response, involving neutrophils (N1), interleukin-22 CD4 T cells, innate lymphoid cells 3 (NCR+ ILC3), iNKT17 cells, and IgG2 B cells[1]. However, some extracellular protozoa can tolerate a TH17 immune response, involving neutrophils (N2), interleukin-17 CD4 T cells, NCR- ILC3, iNKT17 cells, and IgA2 B cells.[1]
- ***Helminths***: Endoparasites such as helminths typically elicit a TH2a immune response, with inflammatory eosinophils (iEOS), interleukin-5/interleukin-4 CD4 T cells, interleukin-25 induced inflammatory innate lymphoid cells 2 (iILC2), tryptase-positive mast cells (MCt), iNKT2 cells, and IgG4 B cells.

6.2.4 IMMUNE RESPONSES AGAINST MAJOR PARASITE GROUPS

Protozoa: Protozoan parasites, such as ***Toxoplasma gondii***, ***Giardia intestinalis***, and ***Cryptosporidium parvum***, can cause chronic and persistent infections because they have evolved multiple mechanisms for evading and resisting specific immunity. The immune response to protozoan infections often involves a TH1 immune response, which includes macrophages, interferon gamma (IFN?) CD4 T cells, innate lymphoid cells 1 (NKp44+ ILC1), CD8 T cells (Effector-Memory4, EM4), invariant natural killer T cells 1 (iNKT1) cells, and immunoglobulin G3 (IgG3) B cells. However, some protozoa can tolerate a TH1-like immune response, which involves macrophages (M2), IFN?/TGF? CD4 T cells, NKp44- ILC1, CD8 T cells (EM3), iNKT1 cells, and IgA1 B cells.

Helminths: Helminths, or worms, are endoparasites that typically elicit a TH2a immune response, with inflammatory eosinophils (iEOS), interleukin-5/interleukin-4 CD4 T cells, interleukin-25 induced inflammatory innate lymphoid cells 2 (iILC2), tryptase-positive mast cells (MCt), iNKT2 cells, and IgG4 B cells [^10^]. This type of immune response is important in limiting parasite numbers and reducing tissue damage caused by the parasites.

Ectoparasites: The host immunity against ectoparasites is typically a TH9 immune response, involving regulatory eosinophils, regulatory basophils, interleukin-9 mast cells (MMC9), thymic stromal lymphopoietin induced innate lymphoid cells 2, interleukin-9 CD4 T cells, iNKT2 cells, and IgA2 B cells. This type of immune response helps to limit the damage associated with ectoparasite infections.

These immune responses, although complex and multifaceted, involve a delicate balance between protective immunity and immunopathology.

The immune system responds to parasites by being greatly influenced by various factors related to the parasite itself, such as where it resides in the host, its size, and the stage of its life cycle. Let us have a look at some examples to illustrate this:

Protozoa: Protozoa are typically microscopic, single-celled organisms that can live and multiply inside your body's cells. Some protozoa, like *Plasmodium* spp. (the causative agent of malaria), change their surface proteins during different stages of their life cycle, which helps them evade the host's immune system. The immune response to protozoa is often a balance between TH1 immune responses, which are typically pro-inflammatory and aim to kill the pathogen, and TH2 responses, which can prevent damage to the host tissue.

Helminths: Helminths are larger, multicellular organisms that can be seen without a microscope when they are adults. They usually live in the intestines, blood vessels, or tissues of the host. Helminths, such as *Schistosoma* spp., can modulate the host's immune response to ensure their survival. They often drive a strong TH2 immune response, which is typically anti-inflammatory and can lead to tissue repair and wound healing. Some helminths can also suppress the host's immune system, helping them to survive for many years in the host.

Ectoparasites: Ectoparasites live on the surface of the host and include organisms like ticks, fleas, and lice. The immune response to ectoparasites often involves inflammation at the site of the bite, as well as itching and pain. Ectoparasites can inject saliva into the host that contains compounds to counteract the host's initial inflammatory response, allowing them to feed without being detected.

6.2.5 KEY IMMUNE EFFECTOR MECHANISMS

Protozoa: Protozoan parasites often elicit a cell-mediated immune response, which involves T helper cells, macrophages, and dendritic cells. One key mechanism is **antibody-mediated killing**, where antibodies produced by B cells bind to antigens on the parasite, marking them for destruction by immune cells. This process is also known as opsonization.

Helminths: In response to helminth infections, the immune system often mounts a TH2 immune response, which involves the production of specific antibodies that can bind to and neutralize the parasites. In addition, eosinophils and mast cells are activated, leading to inflammation and tissue repair. A key feature of the immune response to helminths is the formation of **granulomas**, which are organized structures of immune cells that form around the parasites to isolate them.

Ectoparasites: The immune response to ectoparasites often involves inflammation at the site of the bite, as well as itching and pain. Ectoparasites can inject saliva into the host that contains compounds to counteract the host's initial inflammatory response, allowing them to feed without being detected. In some cases, granulomas may also form in response to ectoparasite infections.

6.2.6 IMMUNOPATHOLOGY AND IMMUNE REGULATION

The immune system plays a crucial role in protecting the body from parasitic infections. However, in some cases, immune responses can lead to negative consequences such as hypersensitivity and immunopathology.

- ***Hypersensitivity***: This refers to an exaggerated or inappropriate immune response that can cause damage to the host. In relation to parasitic infections, hypersensitivity reactions can occur when the immune system overreacts to the presence of the parasite. This can lead to inflammation and tissue damage. An example being, in schistosomiasis, a disease caused by a parasitic worm, the immune system's reaction to the eggs of the parasite can lead to granuloma formation and fibrosis, causing significant damage to the liver and intestines.
- ***Immunopathology***: This refers to the damage caused to body tissues because of an immune response. In the case of parasitic infections, the immune response can sometimes be so strong that it ends up causing more harm than the parasite itself. In the case of some reported malaria cases, the immune response to the *Plasmodium* parasite can lead to the destruction of red blood cells, causing anaemia. In severe cases, the immune response can also cause cerebral malaria, a life-threatening condition characterized by seizures, coma, and other neurological symptoms.

In summary, although the immune system is essential for fighting off parasitic infections, an overactive or misdirected immune response can lead to further complications as stated above, causing significant harm to the host. Therefore, a balanced and well-regulated immune response is crucial for effectively combating parasitic infections without causing undue harm to the host.

6.3 MECHANISMS OF IMMUNE REGULATION AND THEIR ROLE IN CONTROLLING INFLAMMATION AND TISSUE DAMAGE

The immune system is a complex network of cells, tissues, and biochemicals that defends the body against viruses, bacteria, and other pathogens. However, an overactive immune response can lead to inflammation and tissue damage. Therefore, the immune system has several mechanisms to regulate its activity and prevent such damage. Here are some key mechanisms:

- ***Negative feedback loops***: The immune system uses negative feedback loops to regulate its response. When a pathogen is detected, immune cells are sent into a state of activation to fight off the infection. As the pathogen is eliminated, signals are sent to "turn off" the immune response and return the system to a state of balance.

- ***Regulatory T cells (Tregs)***: Tregs are a type of white blood cell that plays a crucial role in maintaining immune homeostasis. They suppress the immune response of other cells to prevent excessive reactions and autoimmunity, a condition where the immune system attacks the body's own cells.
- ***Cytokines***: They are small proteins released by cells that have a specific effect on the interactions and communications between cells. Some cytokines can promote inflammation (pro-inflammatory cytokines like TNF-alpha, IL-1, IL-6), while others can reduce inflammation and promote healing (anti-inflammatory cytokines like IL-10, TGF-beta).
- ***Apoptosis***: This is a process of programmed cell death. When immune cells have served their purpose, they undergo apoptosis (cell death), which helps to prevent an overactive immune response and limit inflammation.
- ***Immunological tolerance***: This is the immune system's ability to differentiate between the body's own cells (self) and foreign cells (non-self). This prevents the immune system from attacking the body's own cells, which could lead to autoimmune diseases.

These mechanisms play a crucial role in controlling inflammation and preventing tissue damage. However, when these regulatory processes fail or are overwhelmed (for example, in chronic inflammation or autoimmune diseases), they can lead to tissue damage and disease. Therefore, understanding and manipulating these regulatory mechanisms is a key focus of many therapeutic strategies for inflammatory and autoimmune diseases.

6.3.1 CO-EVOLUTION AND IMMUNOLOGICAL ADAPTATIONS

There is a dynamic interplay between parasite evasion and host immune adaptation. This interplay, often described as a "molecular arms race," involves the following key processes:

- ***Parasite evasion***: Parasites have evolved various strategies to evade the host's immune system. These include antigenic variation (changing surface proteins to avoid recognition), immune suppression (reducing the host's immune response), and hiding in immune-privileged sites (areas of the body where the immune response is limited, like the brain).

- ***Host immune adaptation***: The host's immune system, in turn, adapts to these evasion strategies. This can involve the production of a broader range of antibodies to recognize different antigens, the activation of different immune pathways to counteract immune suppression, and the development of mechanisms to target parasites in immune-privileged sites.
- ***Co-evolution***: Over time, this dynamic interplay can lead to co-evolution, where changes in the parasite's evasion strategies drive changes in the host's immune adaptations, and vice versa. This can result in a continual cycle of adaptation and counter-adaptation, shaping the evolution of both the host and the parasite.

This dynamic interplay is crucial in determining the outcome of infections. However, it also presents challenges, as the continual evolution of parasites can render treatments ineffective over time, necessitating ongoing research and adaptation of treatment strategies.

Discuss examples of co-evolutionary arms races between specific parasites and hosts.

To shed more light on the complexity of this co-evolutionary "arms race," there are a few examples to peruse:

- ***Malaria and humans***: The *Plasmodium* parasite, which causes malaria, and humans have been engaged in a co-evolutionary arms race for thousands of years. One example of this is the emergence of sickle cell trait in human populations where malaria is prevalent. Sickle cell trait provides some resistance to malaria, demonstrating an adaptation to the parasite. On the other hand, the *Plasmodium* parasite has evolved complex life cycles and antigenic variation to evade the human immune system.
- ***HIV and humans***: HIV, the virus that causes AIDS, has a high mutation rate that allows it to rapidly evolve and escape the immune response. In response, the human immune system has evolved various mechanisms to recognize and attack the virus. For instance, certain human populations have a mutation in the CCR5 receptor (CCR5-delta32) that provides resistance to HIV infection.
- ***Rabbits and myxoma virus***: In the 1950s, the myxoma virus was introduced into Australia to control the rabbit population. Initially, the virus killed a very high percentage of rabbits. However, over time, the rabbits evolved resistance, and the virus evolved to become less virulent, leading to an ongoing co-evolutionary arms race.

6.3.2 POTENTIAL IMPACT OF CO-EVOLUTION ON VACCINE DEVELOPMENT

- ***Antigenic variation***: One of the strategies parasites use to evade the host's immune system is antigenic variation, where they change their surface proteins to avoid recognition. This poses a challenge for vaccine development as the immune system may not recognize the parasite if it has changed its antigens. This is a significant issue in diseases like influenza and HIV, where the virus rapidly mutates and changes its surface proteins.
- ***Immune evasion***: Parasites have evolved various mechanisms to evade the host's immune response, such as suppressing the immune response or hiding in immune-privileged sites. These evasion strategies can make it difficult for a vaccine to elicit a strong and effective immune response.
- ***Strain-specific immunity***: In some cases, the immunity developed against one strain of a parasite does not protect against other strains. This is a challenge in diseases like malaria, where there are multiple species of Plasmodium parasites.
- ***Evolutionary pressure***: Vaccination can exert evolutionary pressure on parasites, potentially leading to the emergence of vaccine-resistant strains. This is a concern in the use of live attenuated vaccines, which contain a weakened form of the pathogen.

In summary, the dynamic and complex nature of host–parasite co-evolution presents both challenges and opportunities for vaccine development. Understanding these interactions can inform the design of more effective vaccines and therapeutic strategies.

6.4 FUTURE DIRECTIONS AND CHALLENGES

Certainly, here are some emerging research areas in parasite immunology:

Immunomodulation: This involves altering the immune response to achieve a desired outcome. Some parasites can modulate the host's immune system to enhance their survival. Understanding these mechanisms can provide insights into the immune system and inform the development of new therapies.

- ***Vaccine development***: Despite the availability of antiparasitic drugs, vaccines remain the most effective way to prevent parasitic infections. However, developing vaccines for parasites is challenging due to their complex life cycles and immune evasion strategies. Current research is focused on identifying protective antigens, understanding the immune responses needed for protection, and developing novel vaccine delivery platforms.

- ***Personalized medicine***: This involves tailoring medical treatment to the individual characteristics of each patient. In the context of parasite immunology, this could involve using genetic or immunological profiling to predict susceptibility to infection, disease severity, or response to treatment. This approach could lead to more effective and targeted treatments for parasitic infections.

These fields are at the cutting edge of parasite immunology, holding great promise for enhancing our knowledge of parasitic diseases and refining their prevention and cure methods.

Controlling parasitic diseases presents several challenges but also opens up new directions for future research. Here are some key points:

6.4.1 CHALLENGES

- ***Drug resistance***: Many parasites have developed resistance to existing antiparasitic drugs, making treatment more difficult.
- ***Vaccine development***: Developing effective vaccines for parasitic diseases is challenging due to the complex life cycles of parasites and their ability to evade the host's immune system.
- ***Access to treatment***: In many parts of the world, especially in low-income countries, access to effective treatment and preventive measures is limited.
- ***Co-infections***: Parasitic diseases often occur in conjunction with other infectious diseases, complicating treatment and prevention efforts.

6.4.2 FUTURE DIRECTIONS

- ***New drug development***: There is a need for new drugs that can effectively treat parasitic diseases and to which parasites have not yet developed resistance.
- ***Improved diagnostics***: Developing more accurate and accessible diagnostic tools can help ensure that parasitic diseases are identified and treated promptly.

- ***Vector control***: Controlling the vectors that transmit parasites, such as mosquitoes for malaria, can be an effective way to prevent parasitic diseases.
- ***Genetic research***: Advances in genetic research could lead to new strategies for controlling parasitic diseases, such as genetically modifying mosquitoes to prevent them from transmitting parasites.
- ***Public health initiatives***: Strengthening public health infrastructure and education can help prevent parasitic diseases and ensure that those affected receive appropriate treatment.

These challenges and future directions highlight the ongoing need for research and innovation in the field of parasitic diseases.

6.5 SUMMARY

- ***Immune responses to parasites***: The immune system plays a crucial role in protecting the body from parasitic infections. However, in some cases, the immune response can lead to negative consequences such as hypersensitivity and immunopathology.
- ***Parasite evasion and host immune adaptation***: Parasites have evolved various strategies to evade the host's immune system. In response, the host's immune system adapts to these evasion strategies. This dynamic interplay is often described as a "molecular arms race" and can lead to co-evolution.
- ***Impact of co-evolution on vaccine development***: Co-evolution between parasites and their hosts can have significant implications for vaccine development. Understanding these interactions can inform the design of more effective vaccines and therapeutic strategies.
- ***Emerging research areas in parasite immunology***: These include immunomodulation, vaccine development, personalized medicine, understanding immune evasion mechanisms, and studying host–parasite co-evolution.
- ***Challenges and Future directions in controlling parasitic diseases***: Challenges include drug resistance, difficulties in vaccine development, access to treatment, and co-infections. Future directions include new drug development, improved diagnostics, vector control, genetic research, and strengthening public health initiatives.

Understanding parasite–host immune interactions is of paramount importance as it not only enhances our knowledge of how our immune system works but also informs the development of effective strategies for the prevention and treatment of parasitic diseases. It is a dynamic and complex field with the potential to significantly impact global health.

FURTHER READING

Brooker, S., & Bundy, D. (2014). Soil-transmitted Helminths (Geohelminths). *Manson's Tropical Diseases*, 1515–1548. https://doi.org/10.1016/B978-0-7020-5101-2.00056-X

Chu Y.-T., Liao M.-T., Tsai K.-W., Lu K.-C., & Hu W.-C. (2023). Interplay of chemokines receptors, toll-like receptors, and host immunological pathways. *Biomedicines*, 11(9), 2384. https://doi.org/10.3390/biomedicines11092384

Donnelly, S. (2022). The immunology of parasite infections: Grand challenges. *Frontiers in Parasitology*, 1, 1069205. https://doi.org/10.3389/fpara.2022.1069205?

Evering, T., & Weiss, L. M. (2006). The immunology of parasite infections in immunocompromised hosts. *Parasite Immunology*, 28(11), 549–565. https://doi.org/10.1111/j.1365-3024.2006.00886.

Field, M. C. (2022). Molecular cellular parasitology: The decades and challenges ahead. *Frontiers in Parasitology*, 1, 963515.

Krüger, T., Schuster, S., & Engstler, M. (2018). Beyond blood: African trypanosomes on the move. *Trends in Parasitology*, 34(12), 1056–1067.

Minciullo, P. & Cascio, A., Isola, S. & Gangemi, S. (2016). Different clinical allergological features of Taenia solium infestation. *Clinical and Molecular Allergy*, 14. https://doi.org/10.1186/s12948-016-0056-x

Moser, W., Schindler, C., & Keiser, J. (2018). Drug combinations against soil-transmitted helminth infections. *Advances in Parasitology*, 103, 91-115. https://doi.org/10.1016/bs.apar.2018.08.002

Reina-San-Martín, B., Cosson, A., & Minoprio, P. (2000). Lymphocyte polyclonal activation: A pitfall for vaccine design against infectious agents. *Parasitology Today*, 16(2), 62–67.

Wen, T. H., Tsai, K. W., Wu, Y. J., Liao, M. T., Lu, K. C., & Hu, W. C. (2021). The framework for human host immune responses to four types of parasitic infections and relevant key JAK/STAT signaling. *International Journal of Molecular Sciences*, 22(24), 13310. https://doi.org/10.3390/ijms22241331

Zhang, K., Jing, X., & Wang, G. (2016). MicroRNAs as regulators of drug abuse and immunity. *Central European Journal of Immunology*, 41(4), 426–434. https://doi.org/10.5114/ceji.2016.6514

7 Parasite–Host–Environment Association

One of the truest tests of integrity is its blunt refusal to be compromised.

Chinua Achebe

CHAPTER OUTLINE

In this chapter, you will explore the dynamic relationship between parasites, their hosts, and the environments in which they thrive. You'll learn how these interactions shape parasite survival, disease transmission, and evolution. This chapter sets the foundation for understanding how parasitic organisms adapt to changing conditions within their hosts and the external world. By the end of this chapter, you will be able to:

- *Understand the Concept of Parasitism*: Learn what parasitism means and how it differs from other biological associations. Examine how parasites evolve from free-living organisms to highly specialized dependent forms.
- *Recognize Levels of Dependence*: Distinguish between free-living parasites, facultative parasites, and total parasites, and understand how metabolic dependence on the host varies among different species.
- *Explore Factors of Dependence*: Discover how parasites rely on their hosts for developmental stimuli, nutrition, digestive enzymes, and maturation control, and understand how these dependencies sustain the parasite's life cycle.
- *Identify Habitats of Parasites*: Examine the various habitats within the host – such as the alimentary canal, blood, tissues, and body cavities – and learn how physicochemical conditions like pH, oxygen, bile, and viscosity influence parasite survival.
- *Understand Environmental Influences*: Analyse how environmental factors shape parasite adaptation, genetic structure, and evolution, with examples from *Plasmodium*, *Trypanosoma*, and other medically important parasites.

DOI: 10.1201/9781003733935-7

- *Study Parasite Niches and Adaptations*: Explore the concept of ecological niches – including food, habitat, and reproductive niches – and how parasites adjust biochemically and structurally to survive in changing host environments.
- *Examine Organ-specific Infections*: Learn which parasites target specific organs such as the brain, liver, lungs, skin, and reproductive organs, and the associated clinical manifestations.
- *Correlate Location with Symptoms, Diagnosis, and Treatment*: Understand how infection site determines symptoms, diagnostic methods, and appropriate treatments, including pharmacological and surgical interventions.
- *Explore the Role of the Environment in Parasite Evolution and Virulence*: Discover how environmental shifts drive genetic adaptation, alter virulence, and affect parasite propagation and host response.
- *Learn Prevention and Control Measures*: Study essential public health strategies – including hygiene, sanitation, vector control, and food and water safety – that help prevent and control parasitic infections.
- *Reflect on Historical Perspectives*: Trace early methods of infection control, including *Tyndallization*, *Salvarsan*, and *Neosalvarsan*, which marked important milestones in parasitology and chemotherapy.

7.1 PARASITISM

Parasitism involves an association between two different species – host and parasite. Most parasites occur as free-living but assume a parasitic existence after contacting a suitable host. Parasites are often in an intimate and continuous association with their hosts. While they may not rapidly destroy their hosts, there may be physiological, immunological, or metabolic interactions that could ultimately result in the survival of either parasite or host, or persistence of both. The association between a parasite and its host is characterized by the level of metabolic dependence.

- When the metabolic dependence on the host is minimal (0%), the parasite is considered free-living (e.g., *Naegleria fowleri* and *Strongyloides stercoralis* existing outside the host).
- When the metabolic dependence is at its peak (100%), the association is regarded as total parasitism (e.g., *Plasmodium* spp. in blood).

- There are other varying levels of metabolic dependence between the extremes, and these are also encountered in nature.

7.2 METABOLIC DEPENDENCE

Parasites depend on their hosts for one or more of the following for survival, replication, and defence:

- ***Developmental stimuli***: Each host environment is equipped with the necessary factors (temperature, pH, oxygen, carbon dioxide, bile, etc.) that are suitable for the establishment of specific parasites. These factors may be essential in stimulating the parasite to develop within the host. For instance, most parasites in the encysted stage utilize high levels of carbon dioxide in the intestines as a signal for excystment, e.g., metacercarial cysts of trematodes and oocysts of coccidia. Many cestodes also use bile as a stimulus for the evagination of the scolex.
- ***Nutritional dependence***: Nutritional supplies may be from the food of the host either before or after digestion, or from the tissues or secretions of the host. *Schistosoma haematobium* in the mesenteric veins of man totally depends on the host for nutrition. *Trypanosoma cruzi*, which lacks the ability to synthesize cholesterol like most parasites, takes up and stores host cholesterol. *Toxoplasma gondii* also utilizes host glucose for intracellular replication.
- ***Digestive enzymes***: Utilization of food from the host is largely dependent on whether or not the parasite can break it down and use the products for growth and differentiation. While many trematodes and nematodes possess the required enzymes to hydrolyse food molecules, some others, such as adult tapeworms, depend on the host's ability to digest carbohydrates, proteins and fats. Adult tapeworms, therefore, utilize the metabolic products from the host.
- ***Control of maturation***: This process often requires a synchronization between the host and the parasite, resulting in the maturation and propagation of the parasite. Hormonal activities within the host may influence the life cycles of some parasites. Mitotic activity of parasites may also follow the circadian rhythm of the host. Additionally, some parasites undergo a multiplication phase leading to an increase in gametocytes, which are released especially during the breeding season of their hosts.

7.3 NICHES, HABITATS, AND ENVIRONMENTS

Niche refers to the unique combination of biotic and abiotic factors which are capable of supporting life. It also describes the interaction an organism has with other species and how that organism fits within its environment. Niches are peculiar to different species, and as such, no two species have the exact same niche. Parasites have a food niche, a habitat niche, a reproductive niche, and physical and chemical niches.

Habitat refers to the place where an organism resides. This includes spaces within the host where a parasite may occupy. For example, the alimentary canal, bloodstream, respiratory system, urinary tract, etc.

Environment consists of all the conditions that surround any living organism. The environment of a parasite living within a vertebrate or invertebrate host may differ from that of a parasite living within the soil.

7.4 THE ALIMENTARY CANAL AS A HABITAT FOR PARASITES

The physicochemical conditions (viscosity, pH, oxygen, and carbon dioxide levels, hydrolysing enzymes, peristaltic movements, host immune responses, etc.) within the alimentary canal of vertebrates generally render it unfavourable for most parasites. These characteristics, therefore, play a critical role in determining the tropism of many parasite species.

a. ***Viscosity***: The viscous film of mucus that lines the gut allows the attachment of many parasites, including cestodes. This close adhesion to the intestinal mucosa is essential for food absorption, diffusion of waste materials, and fertilization.
b. ***pH***: pH varies substantially from site to site, within the gut. While the pH of the mouth ranges from 5.6 to 7.6, the stomach maintains a strongly acidic environment, which limits the survival of most parasites. Many intestinal protozoa exist in an encysted form during passage through the stomach due to the harsh pH. The relatively higher pH of the small and large intestines makes them more conducive to parasite survival.
c. ***Oxygen***: Oxygen levels determine what parasite species occupy a particular site within the gut, as they may either be

aerobic or anaerobic. Flatworms, for instance, exhibit aerobic and anaerobic metabolism depending on the availability of oxygen in their environment. The amount of oxygen available to a parasite may also be affected by the presence of microflora in the immediate vicinity.

d. ***Carbon dioxide***: This gas plays an important role in the metabolism of most parasites. Carbon dioxide is also a necessary factor in the excystment of protozoan and trematode cysts, as well as the hatching of nematode eggs. Parasites can recognize the high level of carbon dioxide within the gut environment for their use.
e. ***Bile***: this is also important for the evagination of cestode scolexes, the excystment of protozoan and trematode cysts, as well as the hatching of helminth eggs.

The mouth, oesophagus, and stomach are the least inhabited sites within the alimentary canal because these environments are often unconducive for most parasites. The most popular habitats, however, are the duodenum, ileum, colon, and the caecum.

- ***Duodenum***: Crypts within the duodenum provide an optimum environment for some protozoa. The high nutritional level of duodenal contents also supports parasite life.
- ***Ileum***: Although the availability of food materials in the ileum is reduced due to absorption, the intestinal cells provide an alternative source of nutrients for some parasites.
- ***Colon and caecum***: Most intestinal parasites are found here because these regions are conducive and comparatively inactive.

7.5 THE BLOOD AS A HABITAT FOR PARASITES

Blood nutrients such as triglycerides, lecithin, cholesterol, amino acids, and glucose are of physiological importance to parasites, which are well adapted to this habitat. The low concentrations of these substances limit the number of parasites that can survive in the blood. For cestodes, the duodenum provides a higher level of nutrition than the blood because they lack a digestive system and are dependent on host nutrients. Conversely, *Schistosoma* and *Plasmodium* spp. have the capacity to metabolize blood cells and plasma solutes for their use.

Blood gases: Oxygen and carbon dioxide are important for the survival of blood parasites. Although the gaseous content of arterial and venous blood differs, carbon dioxide content is remarkably constant and thus may favour parasites with a high CO_2 requirement.

Blood globulins: These are concerned with immune reactions, especially the production of antibodies. The persistence of a parasite within the blood also depends largely on specific immune interactions. The immune status of the host, therefore, may determine the survival rate of parasites in the blood.

7.6 TISSUES AND OTHER HABITATS

Muscle: The function of the human muscle generally makes it an unfavourable site for many parasites. Muscle cells contain high levels of ATP and components such as myoglobin, myosin, actin, creatine, and creatine phosphate. The protozoan *Sarcocystis* and the nematode *Trichinella spiralis* are, however, well adapted to skeletal muscles.

Liver: The liver is rich in accessory growth factors, including iron, vitamins, and plasma proteins. It also has excellent arterial and venous supply with a neutral pH, making it a favourable habitat for tissue parasites and parasites nearby. Its ability to produce bile facilitates the life cycle of many parasites as well. Protozoans and several helminths are the main parasites found in the liver.

Peritoneal cavity: Many larval helminths occur in the body cavity of mammals. The physicochemical properties and cellular constituents of the peritoneal cavity make it suitable for certain parasites to thrive there.

Cerebrospinal fluid: CSF is a dialysate of blood plasma. It contains lower proportions of proteins and antibodies compared to blood. The result is that parasites may persist in the central nervous system even after antibodies have eliminated them from other parts of the body.

7.7 IMPORTANCE OF ENVIRONMENTS IN PARASITE LIFE CYCLES

Parasites are exposed to different environments during their life cycles. Different environments are associated with changes in nutritional and physicochemical conditions, as well as alterations in host factors (microbiota, variable immune responses, metabolic fluctuations, and drug pressure). Nonetheless, most parasites have the ability to adapt to their constantly changing environment.

7.7.1 PARASITE ENVIRONMENTS AND EVOLUTION

Changes in the parasite environment may impact parasite genetic structure, especially if there is constant resistance and adaptation between the parasites and their hosts. This could result in a bidirectional host–parasite co-evolution, which might in turn affect the genetic diversity of both the parasite and host.

Evolution may bring about different parasite species, and more importantly, equip parasite populations with the ability to evade host immunity and rapidly react to alterations in the environmental milieu so as to adapt to new host resources.

Parasites have the ability to sense nutritional and physicochemical changes within their environment and respond appropriately by undergoing biochemical and ultrastructural changes in order to adjust. This usually triggers differentiation, or the next phase of development in the parasite life cycle. For example, hemoflagellates like *Trypanosoma rhodesiense* and *Leishmania mexicana* are able to switch from the nutritionally rich, oxygen-rich, mammalian bloodstream to the nutritionally poor, oxygen-poor insect gut by the synthesis of mitochondria and other associated biochemical processes. A decline in temperature and alteration in the chemical environment causes differentiation into the insect-infective procyclic form of the parasite.

Malaria parasites pass from the vertebrate host to the Anopheles mosquito vector. Within the mosquito host, *Plasmodium* parasites can detect and respond to a fall in temperature, a rise in pH, and the presence of a mosquito-specific factor, xanthurenic acid, which triggers a final differentiation step into male and female gametes.

7.7.2 PARASITE ENVIRONMENTS AND PROPAGATION

The degree of differentiation, the rate of development, or the reproductive capacity of a parasite is dependent on the nutritional value of the particular environment, endocrine behaviour of the host, circadian rhythm, among other factors. Marked differences, however, exist between species. For instance, the egg production of *S. japonicum* is 100 times that of *S. mansoni*, although both species inhabit the portal system of mammals.

7.7.3 PARASITE ENVIRONMENTS AND VIRULENCE

Alterations in the parasite's environment can also have profound effects on characteristics such as virulence. For instance, the asexual blood stage of *Plasmodium* parasites can sense the levels of host nutrient intake and modulate replication and virulence based on nutrient availability.

The sexual stage also responds to variations in the levels of the host lipid lysophosphatidylcholine. Sexual differentiation is suppressed in vitro when lysophosphatidylcholine levels are high. Also, the growth of *Toxoplasma gondii* is substantially inhibited by maintaining the host on a milk diet deficient in p-aminobenzoic acid.

Parasites may also release certain molecules to which the host responds. These molecules often suppress or stimulate host immune responses, downregulate host cell proteins, modify host cell gene expression, or support host cell proliferation. For example, extracellular vesicles released from *Leishmania*-infected macrophages elicit a pro-inflammatory response, induce cytokine production, and thereby modulate disease progression.

Extracellular vesicles released from *Plasmodium*-infected red blood cells can also affect gene expression in endothelial cells and consequently alter barrier properties, leading to vascular dysfunction.

TABLE 7.1 Parasitic Infections by Organ and Tissue Affected

Organ/Tissue Affected	*Parasite Infection*
Brain	• *Naegleria fowleri* • *Taenia solium* • *Echinococcus granulosus* • *Toxoplasma gondii* • *Plasmodium falciparum* • *Schistosoma* spp. • *Acanthamoeba* spp. • *Entamoeba histolytica* • *Trypanosoma* spp. • *Strongyloides stercoralis*

(*Continued*)

TABLE 7.1 (CONTINUED) Parasitic Infections by Organ and Tissue Affected

Organ/Tissue Affected	*Parasite Infection*
Eye	• *Brugia malayi* • *Dirofilaria* spp. • *Ascaris lumbricoides* • *Trichinella* spp. • *Coenurus cerebralis* • *Spirometra* spp. • *Taenia crassiceps* • *Loa loa*
Nasal cavity	• *Ascaris lumbricoides* • *Leishmania* spp.
Oral cavity	• *Entamoeba gingivalis* • *Trichomonas tenax* • *Leishmania* spp. • *Gongylonema pulchrum*
Ear	• *Rhabditis* spp.
Lungs	• *Paragonimus westermani* • *Ascaris lumbricoides* • *Ancylostoma duodenale* • *Necator americanus* • *Schistosoma* spp. • *Strongyloides stercoralis* • *Entamoeba histolytica* • *Leishmania* spp.
Heart	• *Toxoplasma gondii* • *Taenia solium* • *Schistosoma* spp. • *Naegleria fowleri* • *Heterophyes heterophyes* • *Paragonimus westermani* • *Echinococoss granulosus* • *Trypanosoma* spp.
Kidney	• *Dioctophyma renale* • *Echinococcus granulosus* • *Toxoplasma gondii* • *Trichinella spiralis*
Urinary bladder	• *Schistosoma* spp. • *Trichinella spiralis*

(*Continued*)

TABLE 7.1 (CONTINUED) Parasitic Infections by Organ and Tissue Affected

Organ/Tissue Affected	*Parasite Infection*
Liver	• *Cryptosporidium* spp. • *Toxoplasma* spp. • *Ascaris lumbricoides* • *Entamoeba histolytica* • *Trichinella spiralis* • *Clonorchis sinensis*
Spleen	• *Plasmodium falciparum* • *Leishmania* spp. • *Echinococcus granulosus* • *Trichinella spiralis*
Gastrointestinal tract	• *Giardia lamblia* • *Entamoeba histolytica* • *Cryptosporidium* spp. • *Ascaris lumbricoides* • *Trichiuris trichiura* • *Ancylostoma duodenale* • *Necator americanus* • *Hymenolepis* spp. • *Balantidium coli* • *Schistosoma* spp. • *Taenia* spp.
Reproductive organs	• *Trichomonas vaginalis* • *Enterobius vermicularis* • *Schistosoma haematobium* • *Toxoplasma gondii* • *Leishmania* spp.
Skin	• *Sarcoptes scabiei* • *Tunga penetrans* • *Pediculus humanus var. corporis* • *Trypanosoma* spp. • *Leishmania* spp. • *Onchocerca volvulus*
Hair	• *Pediculus humanus var. capitis* • *Pediculus humanus var. pubis* • *Demodex folliculorum*
Nails	• *Tunga penetrans*
Muscles	• *Taenia solium* • *Trichinella spiralis* • *Toxoplasma gondii* • *Brachiola algerae*

(*Continued*)

TABLE 7.1 (CONTINUED) Parasitic Infections by Organ and Tissue Affected

Organ/Tissue Affected	*Parasite Infection*
Joints	• *Giardia lamblia* • *Hymenolepis diminuta* • *Schistosoma* spp. • *Blastocystis hominis* • *Toxocara canis* • *Entameoaba histolytica*
Blood	• *Microfilaria* • *Plasmodium* spp. • *Trypanosoma* spp. • *Leishmania* spp. • *Toxoplasma gondii* • *Babesia* spp.
Lymph	• *Wuchereria bancrofti* • *Brugia* spp. • *Onchocerca volvulus* • *Trypanosoma* spp.

7.7.4 PREVENTION AND CONTROL OF PARASITIC INFECTIONS

As with all things infection related, it is quite difficult to completely eradicate, as factors like human interactions and other mitigating factors are involved.

- ***Wash hands frequently and thoroughly***: Use soap and water for at least 20 seconds, especially before eating, after using the restroom, and after handling animals or their waste.
- ***Shower or bathe regularly***: Maintain good personal hygiene to remove potential parasites and their eggs from your skin.
- ***Practice safe sanitation***: Ensure proper disposal of human waste and avoid contact with untreated sewage, especially in high-risk areas.
- ***Cook food thoroughly***: Ensure proper cooking temperatures (internal temperature) to kill any potential parasites present in meat, fish, or poultry.
- ***Wash fruits and vegetables***: Thoroughly wash all fruits and vegetables before consumption, especially those eaten raw.
- ***Drink safe water***: Consume only bottled or treated water, especially when travelling to areas with high parasitic infection risks.
- ***Avoid undercooked or raw meat***: Refrain from consuming undercooked or raw meat (including seafood) in regions with high parasitic prevalence.

TABLE 7.2 Location of Parasitic Infections, Symptoms, Diagnosis and Treatment

Organ/Tissue Location	*Signs and Symptoms*	*Diagnosis*	*Treatment*
Brain	• Headaches • Seizures • Nausea • Vomiting • Fever • Chills • Itching • Joint pains • Sleepiness • Personality changes • Confusion • Lack of attention to people and surroundings, • Difficulty with balance • Excess fluid around the brain (hydrocephalus)	• Physical examination • Blood tests • Serology • Stool tests • imaging studies (like MRI and CT scans • Biopsies • Spinal tap (lumbar puncture)	• Taking medications such as praziquantel, albendazole, Artemisinin-based combination therapies (ACTs) such as Artemether-Lumefantrine, anti-seizure medications • Surgery • Using corticosteroids • Providing supportive care

(*Continued*)

TABLE 7.2 (CONTINUED) Location of Parasitic Infections, Symptoms, Diagnosis and Treatment

Organ/Tissue Location	*Signs and Symptoms*	*Diagnosis*	*Treatment*
Eye	• Pain in the eye • Sensitivity to light eye redness • Excessive tearing • Blurred vision • Yellow, green or bloody eye discharge • Eyes stuck upon waking up • Swollen eyelids • Loss of vision	• Medical history and examination which may include visual acuity test, slit-lamp examination, funduscopic examination • Imaging test like ultrasound and optical coherence tomography (OCT) • Laboratory tests: These may include blood tests and eye fluid analysis	• Using medications such as pyrimethamine, ivermectin, diethylcarbamazine • Surgery
Nasal Cavity	• Sneezing • Epistaxis • Laryngospasm • Thick mucus nasal discharge • Facial pain • Headache • Dysnoea • Stridor • Passage of worms • Ulcers or sores in the nose	• Medical history and physical examination • Diagnostic tests such as nasal endoscopy, imaging tests, microscopy, blood tests	Surgery Taking antiparasitic medications

(*Continued*)

TABLE 7.2 (CONTINUED) Location of Parasitic Infections, Symptoms, Diagnosis and Treatment

Organ/Tissue Location	*Signs and Symptoms*	*Diagnosis*	*Treatment*
Oral cavity	• Low grade fever • Myaglia • General weakness • Headache • Dizziness • Swollen lymph nodes • Periodontitis • Severe pain • Bad breath • Hypersalivation • Nausea • Vomiting • Cough • Pruritus • Dyspnoea • Sensation of a crawling bug inside the mouth	• Medical history and oral examination • Microscopic examination. • Blood tests • Biopsy	Antiparasitic medications such as metronidazole, albendazole, and ivermectin Pain relief medications Surgery

(Continued)

TABLE 7.2 (CONTINUED) Location of Parasitic Infections, Symptoms, Diagnosis and Treatment

Organ/Tissue Location	*Signs and Symptoms*	*Diagnosis*	*Treatment*
Ear	• Persistent unlocalized ear pain • Swelling • Redness and itching • Unexplained tingling or tickling sensation • Ringing in the ear • Itching	• Otoscopy • Microscopy • Blood tests	• Ear irrigation • Surgery • Antiparasitic medications
Lungs	• Dry Cough • Dyspnoea • Wheezing • Fever • Malaise • Weight loss • Fatigue • Coughing up pink or red phlegm • Shortness of breath • Coughing up worms • Headaches • Hemotysis • Acute pneumonia	• Medical history and physical examination • Imaging tests: X-rays, CT scans, or MRIs. • Sputum analysis • Blood tests • Biopsy	• Antiparasitic medications: Examples include praziquantel for Paragonimiasis, albendazole for Ascariasis, and miltefosine for Leishmaniasis. • Bronchodilators • Corticosteroids

(*Continued*)

TABLE 7.2 (CONTINUED) Location of Parasitic Infections, Symptoms, Diagnosis and Treatment

Organ/Tissue Location	*Signs and Symptoms*	*Diagnosis*	*Treatment*
Heart	• Fever • Fatigue • Chest pains • Shortness of breath • Palpitations • Swollen lymph nodes • Night sweats • Skin rash • Joint pain or muscle aches	• Medical history and physical examination • Blood tests • Imaging tests: Examples echocardiograms, chest X-rays, or CT scans • Biopsy	• Antiparasitic medications such as benznidazole, nifurtimox, pentamidine, suramin, pyrimethamine and sulfadiazine • Surgery
Kidney	• Blood in urine • Cloudy or foamy urine • Frequent urination • Lower back pain • Fever and chills • Fatigue • High blood pressure • Abdominal pain • Nausea and vomiting • Swollen legs or ankles	• Travel history and medical history • Blood tests • Urinalysis • Imaging tests: X-rays, ultrasounds, or CT scans • Kidney biopsy	• Taking medications like Praziquantel, Artimesinin-based combination therapies, Albendazole, diethylcarbamazine (DEC), Benznidazole • Surgery

(*Continued*)

TABLE 7.2 (CONTINUED) Location of Parasitic Infections, Symptoms, Diagnosis and Treatment

Organ/Tissue Location	*Signs and Symptoms*	*Diagnosis*	*Treatment*
Urinary bladder	• Frequent urination • Painful urination • Blood in the urine • Pelvic pain • Cloudy or bloody urine • Bedwetting • Fever	Urine analysis and microscopy Medical history and physical examination Imaging tests: X-rays, ultrasounds, or CT scans	Antiparasitic drugs like praziquantel, or metronidazole
Liver	• Fever • Fatigue • Abdominal pain • Nausea and vomiting • Loss of appetite • Jaundice • Dark urine • Pale stools • Itchy skin • Weight loss	• Medical history and physical examination • Blood tests • Imaging tests like ultrasound, CT scans, or MRIs • Stool examination • Biopsy	• Taking medications like Albendazole, Praziquantel, Nitazoxanide, Metronidazole • Supportive care • Dietary modification • Surgery

(*Continued*)

TABLE 7.2 (CONTINUED) Location of Parasitic Infections, Symptoms, Diagnosis and Treatment

Organ/Tissue Location	*Signs and Symptoms*	*Diagnosis*	*Treatment*
Spleen	• Fever • Fatigue • Upper left abdominal pain • Enlarged spleen • Loss of appetite • Early satiety • Weight loss • Pale skin • General malaise	• Medical history and physical examination. • Blood tests • Imaging techniques like ultrasound, CT scans, or MRIs	Antimalarial medications Surgery
Gastrointestinal tract	• Diarrhoea, dysentery • Constipation • Stomach cramps • Abdominal pain • Vomiting • Dehydration • Headache • Dizziness or fainting • Loss of appetite • Fatigue • Low blood pressure • Low grade fever • Weight loss, particularly in cases that last 2 to 4 weeks	• Medical history and physical examination • Stool examination • Blood tests • Imaging tests such as X-rays, ultrasounds, or endoscopies	• Taking medications such as Albendazole or Metronidazole, Mebendazole, Pyrantel pamoate, Praziquantel, Nitazoxanide • Hydration • Dietary modifications • Taking mineral or vitamin supplements

(*Continued*)

TABLE 7.2 (CONTINUED) Location of Parasitic Infections, Symptoms, Diagnosis and Treatment

Organ/Tissue Location	*Signs and Symptoms*	*Diagnosis*	*Treatment*
Reproductive organs	• Unusual vaginal or penile discharge • Itching, burning or soreness • Pain during sex • Vaginal bleeding outside of menstruation • Painful urination • Pelvic pain or lower abdominal pain • Frequent urination • Swollen lymph nodes in the groin area • Skin rash or sores • Fever or chills	• Medical history and physical exam • Swabs of vaginal or urethral discharge • Urine samples • Blood tests to identify specific antibodies or parasites • Imaging tests	• Medications like Metronidazole Albendazole, Praziquantel • Anti-itch or anti-inflammatory medications • Treating sexual partners simultaneously • Supportive care • Rarely, surgery

(*Continued*)

TABLE 7.2 (CONTINUED) Location of Parasitic Infections, Symptoms, Diagnosis and Treatment

Organ/Tissue Location	*Signs and Symptoms*	*Diagnosis*	*Treatment*
Skin	• Intense itching • Rash • Burrows or tracks • Redness or swelling • Ulcers or open sores • Thickening of the skin • Hair loss • Visible parasites or larvae • Secondary bacterial infection • Fever or chills	• Skin examination • Skin scraping or biopsy • Blood tests	• Permethrin cream is the standard treatment, often requiring a single application. • Crotamiton cream or lotion • Ivermectin (in oral form for severe cases). • Using antihistamines or soothing lotions can help relieve itching. • Thoroughly washing clothes, bedding, and towels in hot water to prevent reinfection. • Antihistamines for itch relief. • Combing • Surgical removal • Use of antibiotics

(*Continued*)

TABLE 7.2 (CONTINUED) Location of Parasitic Infections, Symptoms, Diagnosis and Treatment

Organ/Tissue Location	*Signs and Symptoms*	*Diagnosis*	*Treatment*
Hair	• Itching • Scalp sores • Hair loss • Swollen lymph nodes • Irritability • Poor sleep • Visible parasites	• Visual examination • Microscopy	• Over the counter (OTC) medicated shampoos or lotions often containing permethrin or malathion • Wet combing • Oral medications: In severe cases, ivermectin tablets are prescribed
Muscles	• Muscle pain • Muscle weakness • Muscle fatigue • Swelling • Redness • Tenderness • Fever • Fatigue • Weight loss • Skin rash	• Medical history and physical examination. • Blood tests • Imaging tests: X-rays, CT scans, or MRIs • Muscle biopsy	• Surgery • Physical therapy

(Continued)

TABLE 7.2 (CONTINUED) Location of Parasitic Infections, Symptoms, Diagnosis and Treatment

Organ/Tissue Location	*Signs and Symptoms*	*Diagnosis*	*Treatment*
Joints	• Joint pain • Joint swelling • Joint stiffness • Joint redness • Joint warmth • Joint tenderness • Fever • Fatigue • Muscle weakness • Skin rash	• Medical history and physical examination • Blood tests • Imaging tests: X-rays, ultrasounds, or MRIs • Joint aspiration • Biopsy	• Medications such as Albendazole, • Praziquantel, Ivermectin • Combination therapy • Pain management using medications like NSAIDs (nonsteroidal anti-inflammatory drugs). • Physical therapy • Surgery
Blood	• Fever • Fatigue • Anaemia • Chills. • Headache • Muscle aches and pains • Nausea and vomiting • Weight loss • *Enlarged spleen* • *Skin rash*	• Medical history and physical examination • Blood tests • Microscopy • Imaging tests: X-rays, ultrasounds, or CT scans	• Antimalarials • Antiprotozoal drugs • Anthelmintics. • Supportive care • Blood transfusions • Surgery

(*Continued*)

TABLE 7.2 (CONTINUED) Location of Parasitic Infections, Symptoms, Diagnosis and Treatment

Organ/Tissue Location	*Signs and Symptoms*	*Diagnosis*	*Treatment*
Lymph	• Swollen lymph nodes • Fever • Fatigue • Pain • Skin rash • Loss of appetite • Night sweats • Chills • Muscle aches and pains • Weight loss	Blood tests Physical examination Imaging tests (ultrasound, X-ray) Eye tests Skin biopsy Identification of worms under the skin	Mass drug administration (MDA) with medication like diethylcarbamazine (DEC), Ivermectin, albendazole Using antihistamines Supportive care like compression stockings and lymphedema management

- ***Wear shoes***: Wear shoes, especially sandals or closed-toed shoes, when outdoors in areas with potential parasite transmission, like soil or stagnant water.
- ***Minimize contact with vectors***: Avoid contact with potential vectors like mosquitoes, tsetse flies, or sandflies. Use insect repellents containing DEET, picaridin, or IR3535 and wear protective clothing when necessary.
- ***Maintain clean surroundings***: Keep your living space and surroundings clean and free of potential breeding grounds for parasites, such as stagnant water or rubbish.
- ***Treat pets regularly***: Regularly treat pets (dogs and cats) with vet-recommended medication to prevent them from harbouring and transmitting parasites to humans.
- ***Seek medical advice before travelling***: Consult a healthcare professional before travelling to regions with high parasitic infection risks. Discuss recommended vaccinations, medications, and preventive measures.
- ***Be aware of local risks***: Research the specific parasitic infections prevalent in your travel destination and take appropriate precautions.
- ***Carry necessary medication***: If prescribed by a doctor, carry antimalarial medication or other preventive medications during your travel.
- ***Maintain a healthy immune system***: Practice healthy habits like a balanced diet, regular exercise, and adequate sleep to strengthen your immune system and fight off infections.

Tyndallization – A historical method for sterilizing substances, typically food and liquids, by using repeated cycles of heating and incubation.

Salvarsan – also known as Arsphenamine and compound 606, was the first effective treatment for several parasitic diseases including syphilis and African trypanosomiasis.

Neosalvarsan – a synthetic chemotherapeutic drug used in the early 20th century, primarily for treating syphilis. Developed by Paul Ehrlich in 1912.

7.8 DEFINITION

Peritoneal cavity the fluid-filled space inside the abdomen that surrounds and cushions the organs (like the stomach, intestines, and liver).

FURTHER READING

Brooker, S. & Bundy, D. (2014). Soil-transmitted Helminths (Geohelminths). *Manson's Tropical Diseases*, 1515–1548. https://doi.org/10.1016/B978-0-7020-5101-2.00056-X

Field, M. C. (2022). Molecular cellular parasitology: The decades and challenges ahead. *Frontiers in Parasitology*, 1, 963515.

Gottstein, B. (2001). Animal models in parasitology. *Animal Testing in Infectiology*, 9, 31–44.

Krüger, T., Schuster, S., & Engstler, M. (2018). Beyond blood: African trypanosomes on the move. *Trends in Parasitology*, 34(12), 1056–1067.

Mathison, B. A., & Pritt, B. S. (2022). Parasites of the gastrointestinal tract. In N. Rezaei (Ed.), *Encyclopedia of infection and immunity* (pp. 136–203). Elsevier.

Olano, J. P., Weller, P. F., Guerrant, R. L., & Walker, D. H. (2011). Principles of parasitism: Host–parasite interactions. *Tropical Infectious Diseases: Principles, Pathogens and Practice*, 1–7. https://doi.org/10.1016/B978-0-7020-3935-5.00001-X

Poulin, R., & Randhawa, H. S. (2015). Evolution of parasitism along convergent lines: from ecology to genomics. *Parasitology*, 142(S1), S6–S15. https://doi.org/10.1017/S003118201300167

Reina-San-Martín, B., Cosson, A., & Minoprio, P. (2000). Lymphocyte polyclonal activation: A pitfall for vaccine design against infectious agents. *Parasitology Today*, 16(2), 62–67.

8 Clinical Manifestations of Parasitic Diseases

The energy or active exercise of the mind constitutes life.

Aristotle

CHAPTER OUTLINE

In this chapter, you will explore the diverse ways parasitic infections present in the human body and understand how the interaction between parasites and their hosts leads to disease. Get ready to examine how different groups of parasites – from protozoa to helminths – cause distinct clinical symptoms, and how host, parasite, and environmental factors influence the outcome of infection. By the end of this chapter, you will be able to:

- *Understand the Pathophysiology of Parasitic Infections*: Explore how parasites cause disease through direct tissue damage, immune responses, and toxin production, and how these mechanisms vary among parasite groups.
- *Examine Sarcodine Infections*: Learn how *Entamoeba histolytica* and related parasites invade the intestinal wall, causing ulceration, dysentery, and liver abscesses, and how host immunity contributes to these outcomes.
- *Study Ciliophoran Infections*: Discover how *Balantidium coli* attaches to intestinal tissues, leading to mucoid diarrhoea, ulceration, and systemic complications, especially in immunocompromised individuals.
- *Explore Mastigophoran Infections*: Understand the diseases caused by flagellated parasites such as *Leishmania* and *Trypanosoma*, and the resulting cutaneous lesions, neurological symptoms, and cardiac complications.
- *Investigate Apicomplexan Infections*: Analyse how intracellular parasites like *Plasmodium* and *Toxoplasma* cause cyclic fevers, anaemia, organ failure, and neurological disorders through specialized invasion mechanisms.
- *Understand Cestode Infections*: Learn how tapeworms and their larval stages affect the gastrointestinal system and other organs, producing abdominal discomfort, nutrient loss, seizures, and intestinal obstruction.

DOI: 10.1201/9781003733935-8

- *Recognize Trematode Infections*: Examine how flukes damage tissues mechanically and chemically, leading to hepatobiliary disease, pulmonary symptoms, haematuria, and fibrosis.
- *Describe Nematode Infections*: Study how roundworms cause nutritional deficiencies, inflammation, and obstruction through their migration and feeding behaviour.
- *Correlate Life Cycle Stages with Disease Symptoms*: Understand how different life cycle stages – invasion, migration, reproduction, and transmission – correspond to changes in symptom timing and severity.
- *Analyse Host, Parasite, and Environmental Factors*: Explore how genetics, immunity, parasite virulence, co-infections, and environmental conditions shape the clinical presentation of parasitic diseases.
- *Appreciate Clinical Implications*: Learn how recognizing distinct symptom patterns aids in diagnosis, differential interpretation, and improved patient management.

8.1 PATHOPHYSIOLOGY OF PARASITIC INFECTIONS

Pathophysiology refers to the study of the functional changes that occur in the body as a result of a disease or abnormal condition. The pathophysiology of parasitic infections involves complex interactions between the parasite and its host, leading to various disease conditions.

These interactions can be direct, where the parasite directly affects host cells or tissues, or indirect, where molecules from the parasites trigger a cascade of events in the host that result in disease symptoms.

8.1.1 PATHOPHYSIOLOGY OF INFECTIONS ASSOCIATED WITH SARCODINE PARASITES

Sarcodine parasites like *Entamoeba histolytica* primarily affect the gastrointestinal tract, particularly the large intestine. These parasites can also affect the lungs, liver, and the urinary tract.

Through adhesion and invasion of the host's epithelial cells, sarcodine parasites cause the formation of ulcers and abscesses in the intestine.

This invasion can cause severe abdominal pain, diarrhoea, and dysentery. Also, the release of enzymes contributing to the damage and inflammation observed in infections like amoebic dysentery, coupled with the host's immune response, plays a crucial role in the pathophysiology of sarcodine infections.

Some clinical manifestations of diseases caused by organisms in the phylum Sarcodina include violent diarrhoea, blood and mucus in stools, dehydration, and severe abdominal cramps.

Other presentations include chills, fever, headache, blocked nose and altered taste and smell.

- Stiff neck
- Kernig's sign, often leading to death within 4–5 days after onset
- Anaemia
- Flatulence
- Abdominal distention
- Steatorrhoea with foul-smell
- Bulky stools
- Anorexia
- Nausea
- Weight loss
- Creamy greenish-yellow discharge
- Itchy and burning sensation

In rare cases, the parasite can also travel to the liver, causing amoebic liver abscess.

8.1.2 PATHOPHYSIOLOGY OF INFECTIONS ASSOCIATED WITH CILIOPHORAN PARASITES

Ciliophorans like Trichodinidae attach firmly to their host's epithelial cells using their adhesive disc or hold-fast organ. The fixed attachment of the parasite can disrupt the host's tissues leading to clinical manifestations.

The host's immune response to the presence of ciliophorans can lead to inflammation and further tissue damage, further aggravating the severity of the disease.

Balantidium coli is the only ciliophoran parasite known to infect humans, causing balantidiasis.

Clinical manifestations of diseases caused by organisms in phylum Ciliophoran include abdominal pain and diarrhoea (which can be bloody or mucoid), nausea, vomiting, and weight loss. It also includes dysentery-like symptoms with frequent, watery stools, ulceration, and inflammation of the intestinal lining, which can lead to perforation.

In severe cases, the infection can spread beyond the intestines to cause liver abscesses, peritonitis, and even death.

Balantidiasis is considered an opportunistic infection, meaning it primarily affects individuals with weakened immune systems, such as those with HIV/AIDS, malnutrition, or other underlying medical conditions.

8.1.3 PATHOPHYSIOLOGY OF INFECTIONS ASSOCIATED WITH MASTIGOPHORAN PARASITES

The pathophysiology of mastigophoran parasites involves a complex interplay of tissue invasion, immune evasion, toxin production, and indirect mechanisms that contribute to the development and progression of the associated diseases.

Mastigophoran parasites can invade and damage various tissues in the human body. For example, *Leishmania* spp. can cause cutaneous, mucocutaneous, and visceral leishmaniasis by infecting and damaging the skin, mucous membranes, and internal organs respectively.

Trypanosoma brucei causes African trypanosomiasis (sleeping sickness) by invading the central nervous system and brain.

Some mastigophoran parasites produce toxins or other pathogenic factors such as proteases that contribute to the clinical manifestations of the disease.

Clinical manifestations of diseases caused by organisms in phylum Mastigophora include solitary or multiple, dry, ulcerating papules on skin, fever, ulceration and destruction of the nasal septum, palate, pharynx, and larynx (known as espundia). There is also weight loss, hepatosplenomegaly, pancytopenia, headaches, joint pains, confusion, poor coordination, disruption of the sleep-wake cycle, heart failure, arrhythmias, megaoesophagus or megacolon, urethral discharge in men, vaginal discharge, itching, and irritation in women.

The clinical manifestations vary depending on the specific mastigophoran parasite causing the disease or infection.

8.1.4 PATHOPHYSIOLOGY OF INFECTIONS ASSOCIATED WITH APICOMPLEXAN PARASITES

The pathophysiology of Apicomplexan parasites is characterized by their obligate intracellular lifestyle, specialized motility and invasion mechanisms, unique cytoskeletal structures, replication and proliferation within host cells, and strategies to evade the host's immune system, all of which contribute to their ability to cause significant morbidity and mortality in humans and animals.

Apicomplexan parasites can only replicate and survive inside the host's cells. The presence of specialized organelles like rhoptries, micronemes, a specialized cytoskeleton, including the apical polar ring, subpellicular microtubules, dense granules and the use of a unique form of motility called "helical gliding" that allows them to invade and establish themselves within the host cells.

Once inside the host cell, Apicomplexan parasites can replicate and proliferate, leading to the destruction of the host cell and the release of new parasites to infect other cells.

Clinical manifestations of diseases caused by organisms in phylum Apicomplexa include fever, malaise, vomiting, headaches, jaundiced skin, seizures, coma, death, chronic anaemia, chills, fatigue, haemolytic anaemia, diarrhoea, abdominal pain, and malabsorption.

The clinical manifestations of Apicomplexan diseases can range from mild symptoms like fever and malaise to severe, life-threatening complications such as organ failure, seizures, and death, depending on the specific parasite involved and the immune status of the host.

8.1.5 PATHOPHYSIOLOGY OF INFECTIONS ASSOCIATED WITH CESTODE PARASITES

Cestoidean parasites have a complex pathophysiology in humans and animals. They are well adapted to their hosts, and adult tapeworms often cause few symptoms and rarely cause serious pathology.

The adult tapeworms attach to the intestinal wall, feed on the nutrients in the host's intestine, and disrupt normal digestion, which leads to the observation of signs and symptoms.

However, larval cestodes that develop in organs or tissues outside the gut can be far more pathogenic.

Clinical manifestations of diseases caused by organisms in phylum Cestoda include abdominal pain, nausea, vomiting, appetite loss, weight loss, moderate eosinophilia, diarrhoea, increased appetite, constipation, and bloating.

In severe cases, intestinal perforation or aspiration of expelled proglottids can occur. Other symptoms that occur in this phase include headaches, dizziness, seizures, sensory deficits, involuntary movements, brain system dysfunction in children and ocular cysts.

8.1.6 PATHOPHYSIOLOGY OF INFECTIONS ASSOCIATED WITH TREMATODE PARASITES

Trematodes can cause tissue damage in the host organism through mechanical and chemical means. The parasites attach to the walls of organs, such as the intestine, liver, lungs, or bile ducts, leading to physical damage and inflammation.

In infections like schistosomiasis, the eggs of the schistosomes can become trapped in tissues, leading to granulomatous inflammatory reactions. In some cases, the presence of trematodes can lead to obstruction of organs or ducts. For example, liver flukes like *Opisthorchis viverrini* can cause inflammation and obstruction in the bile duct, leading to symptoms like abdominal pain and jaundice.

Larval migration can cause damage to tissues and trigger inflammatory responses contributing to pathogenesis.

The symptoms of trematode infections are often related to the location of the parasites in the body.

Clinical manifestations of diseases caused by organisms in phylum Trematoda include abdominal pain, diarrhoea, indigestion, changes in appetite, chronic cough, chest pain, shortness of breath, liver inflammation, jaundice, colic pain, liver cirrhosis, terminal haematuria, dysuria, frequent urination, seizures, headaches, mental confusion, fatigue, weakness, and anaemia.

8.1.7 *PATHOPHYSIOLOGY OF INFECTIONS ASSOCIATED WITH NEMATODE PARASITES*

Nematodes can cause tissue damage in the host through their feeding activities and migration. Adult worms can attach to the intestinal mucosa, leading to mechanical damage and inflammation.

In hypersensitized individuals, nematode infections can trigger allergic reactions, often associated with larval migration through tissues.

Nematodes can interfere with the absorption of proteins, fats, and carbohydrates in the intestines, leading to nutritional deficiencies. This can be particularly problematic in individuals with heavy worm burdens or malnutrition.

Large numbers of worms can form a bolus and cause intestinal obstruction. In severe cases, migrating worms can perforate the intestines, leading to peritonitis and other complications. Larval nematodes that migrate through tissues to complete their life cycle can cause tissue damage, inflammation, and severe disease if they end up in the wrong organ.

Clinical manifestations of diseases caused by nematodes include abdominal discomfort, nausea, vomiting, weight loss, malabsorption of nutrients, diarrhoea, intestinal obstruction, pneumonitis, cough, low-grade fever, and eosinophilia.

8.2 IMPACT OF PARASITE LIFE CYCLES ON SYMPTOMS OF DISEASES

The correlation between the life cycle stages of parasitic organisms and the timing and severity of symptoms is crucial in understanding the clinical presentation of parasitic diseases.

The timing and severity of symptoms are often influenced by the specific life cycle stages of the parasite within the host's body. The life cycle stages of parasitic organisms can impact the timing and severity of symptoms through:

- ***Invasion and initial development***: Symptoms may be absent or mild during the initial stages of invasion and development of the parasite within the host's body. This is because the parasite is establishing itself and may not yet be causing significant damage or triggering an immune response.

- ***Multiplication and migration***: As the parasite multiplies and migrates within the host's body, symptoms may start to manifest. Migration of larvae or adult parasites through tissues can lead to tissue damage, inflammation, and the onset of symptoms such as fever, pain, and organ dysfunction.
- ***Reproductive stage***: During the reproductive stage of the parasite, symptoms may worsen as the parasite produces offspring or releases infective stages into the host's tissues or bloodstream. This can lead to an increase in parasite load and exacerbation of symptoms.
- ***Transmission stage***: When the parasite reaches a stage where it can be transmitted to another host, symptoms may peak as the parasite prepares for transmission. This stage may coincide with the release of infective stages into the environment or the host's bodily fluids, leading to a surge in symptoms.
- ***Cyclic symptoms***: Some parasites exhibit cyclic symptoms that coincide with specific stages of their life cycle. For example, in malaria caused by *Plasmodium* parasites, symptoms like fever occur in cycles corresponding to the release of merozoites from infected red blood cells.

Understanding the correlation between the life cycle stages of parasitic organisms and the timing and severity of symptoms is essential for diagnosing and treating parasitic diseases effectively.

8.3 FACTORS THAT INFLUENCE CLINICAL PRESENTATION OF PARASITIC DISEASES

8.3.1 HOST FACTORS

- ***Genetic polymorphisms***: Variations in genes encoding proteins involved in immune function, cell adhesion, and other processes can affect an individual's susceptibility, pathogenesis, and disease severity.
- ***Immune response***: The host's immune response, including the production of antibodies and the activation of immune cells, can modulate the severity of parasitic infections. For example, individuals with compromised immune systems, such as those with HIV/AIDS, are more susceptible

to opportunistic parasites like *Cryptosporidium* spp. and *Giardia lamblia*.

- ***Age and prior exposure***: Factors like age and previous exposure to the parasite can influence the clinical manifestations, with children and those without prior exposure being more susceptible to severe disease.
- ***Ethnicity and genetic background***: Differences in genetic and ethnic backgrounds may contribute to variations in host-parasite interactions and disease outcomes.

8.3.2 PARASITE FACTORS

- ***Parasite species and strain***: Different species and strains of parasites can have varying pathogenic potential and lead to distinct clinical presentations.
- ***Parasite biomass and virulence***: The total parasite burden, as well as the virulence factors expressed by the parasite, can influence the severity of the disease.
- ***Parasite life cycle and migration***: The specific stage of the parasite's life cycle and its ability to migrate through different tissues can impact the clinical manifestations.

8.3.3 EXTERNAL FACTORS

- ***Environmental conditions***: Factors like climate, geography, and sanitation can affect the transmission and prevalence of parasitic infections, which in turn can influence the clinical presentation.
- ***Co-infections***: The presence of other infections, such as bacterial or viral co-infections, can modulate the host's immune response and the severity of the parasitic disease.
- ***Access to healthcare***: Timely diagnosis and appropriate treatment can significantly impact the clinical course and outcomes of parasitic diseases.
- ***Antibiotic use***: Antibiotic use can influence the clinical presentation of parasitic diseases by altering the gut microbiome and potentially leading to the overgrowth of opportunistic parasites.
- ***Public health measures***: Public health measures like sanitation, hygiene, and vector control can significantly influence the prevalence and severity of parasitic diseases. For example, improved sanitation and hygiene can reduce the risk of waterborne parasites like Giardia.

8.4 DEFINITIONS

Ulcers *are open sores or breaks in the skin or the lining of an organ, such as the stomach or intestines.*

Abscess *is a localized collection of pus within a tissue, organ, or confined space in the body. It forms as a result of infection, usually bacterial, causing tissue breakdown and an inflammatory response.*

Kernig's sign *is a physical examination test used to help diagnose meningitis, an infection of the membranes covering the brain and spinal cord.*

Anorexia *is a medical term meaning loss of appetite or inability to eat. It can occur as a symptom of illness or other conditions.*

Arrhythmias *are irregular heartbeats caused by disturbances in the heart's electrical system. They can make the heart beat too fast, too slow, or irregularly.*

Cytoskeleton *is a network of protein fibres inside a cell that gives the cell its shape, strength, and the ability to move.*

Nausea *is the uneasy sensation in the stomach that often comes before vomiting*

Granulomatous inflammation *is a specific type of chronic inflammation characterized by the formation of granulomas, which are small clusters of immune cells called macrophages*

Pneumonitis *is inflammation or irritation of the lung tissue, often caused by an immune response to inhaled irritants such as chemicals, moulds, dust, or allergens.*

FURTHER READING

Argy, N., Kendjo, E., Augé-Courtoi, C., Cojean, S., Clain, J., Houzé, P., Thellier, M., Hubert, V., Deloron, P., & Houzé, S. (2017). Influence of host factors and parasite biomass on the severity of imported plasmodium falciparum malaria. *PLoS One,* 12(4), e0175328. https://doi.org/10.1371/journal.pone.0175328

Auld, S. K. J. R. & Tinsley, M. C. (2015). The evolutionary ecology of complex lifecycle parasites: Linking phenomena with mechanisms. *Heredity*, 114(2), 125–132. https://doi.org/10.1038/hdy.2014.84

Baker, D. G. (2019). Parasitic diseases. *The Common Marmoset in Captivity and Biomedical Research*, 2019, 289–303. https://doi.org/10.1016/B978-0-12-811829-0.00017-0

Cross, J. H. (1996). Enteric nematodes of humans. In S. Baron (Ed.), *Medical microbiology* (4th ed.). University of Texas Medical Branch at Galveston. http://www.ncbi.nlm.nih.gov/books/NBK8261/

Doughty, B. L. (1996). Schistosomes and other trematodes. In S. Baron (Ed.), *Medical microbiology* (4th ed.). University of Texas Medical Branch at Galveston. http://www.ncbi.nlm.nih.gov/books/NBK8037/

Heyneman, D. (1996). "Cestodes." In S. Baron (Ed.), *Medical microbiology* (4th ed.). University of Texas Medical Branch. http://www.ncbi.nlm.nih.gov/books/NBK8399/

Hommel, M. (1996). [Physiopathology of protozoan infections]. *Comptes Rendus Des Seances De La Societe De Biologie Et De Ses Filiales*, 190(4), 341–355.

Kiani, H., Haghighi, A., Rostaml, A., Azargashb, E., Tabaei, S. J. S., Solgi, A., & Zebardast, N. (2016). Prevalence, risk factors and symptoms associated to intestinal parasite infections among patients with gastrointestinal disorders in Nahavand, Western Iran. *Revista Do Instituto de Medicina Tropical de São Paulo*, 58, 42. https://doi.org/10.1590/S1678-9946201658042

Physiopedia. (2024). Parasitic infections. https://www.physio-pedia.com/Parasitic_Infections

SlideShare. (2016). Subphylum mastigophora. https://www.slideshare.net/NoeMendez9/subphylum-mastigophora.

Sorobetea, D., Svensson-Frej, M., & Grencis, R. (2018). Immunity to gastrointestinal nematode infections. *Mucosal Immunology*, 11(2), 304–315. https://doi.org/10.1038/mi.2017.113

"Taenia Solium." In Wikipedia, 8 May 2024. https://en.wikipedia.org/w/index.php?title=Taenia_solium&oldid=1222868447

9 Laboratory Methods for the Detection of Parasitic Infections

Keep your face to the sunshine and you cannot see a shadow.

Helen Keller

CHAPTER OUTLINE

In this chapter, you will explore the fundamental laboratory techniques used to identify parasitic infections. You'll gain practical insights into specimen collection, diagnostic methods, and modern technologies that ensure accurate detection and management of parasitic diseases. Get ready to develop the essential skills and knowledge every parasitologist and medical laboratory professional must master. By the end of this chapter, you will be able to:

- *Understand Diagnostic Approaches*: Explore the overall diagnostic strategies in parasitology, including microscopy, serology, and molecular methods, and learn when to apply each for effective disease detection.
- *Identify Specimens for Diagnosis*: Recognize the various types of clinical specimens used in parasitology – such as stool, blood, urine, and tissue – and understand how specimen choice depends on the suspected infection.
- *Master Specimen Collection and Preservation*: Learn best practices for specimen collection, handling, transport, and storage, ensuring reliability and accuracy in test results.
- *Explore Microscopic Examination Techniques*: Delve into basic and advanced microscopy, including wet mounts, stained preparations, and blood film examinations for detecting parasites.
- *Apply Concentration and Recovery Methods*: Study sedimentation, flotation, and quantification techniques used to concentrate and identify parasites in clinical samples.
- *Understand Culture and Histopathology*: Examine the role of culture, animal inoculation, and tissue biopsy in detecting difficult-to-identify parasites.

DOI: 10.1201/9781003733935-9

- *Investigate Serological and Immunological Tests*: Gain insight into ELISA, rapid diagnostic tests (RDTs), and immunoblot assays for detecting parasite antigens and antibodies.
- *Discover Molecular Diagnostic Techniques*: Understand how PCR, real-time PCR, and isothermal methods (LAMP) revolutionize parasitic diagnosis through sensitivity and specificity.
- *Recognize Imaging and Modern Diagnostic Tools*: Explore how ultrasound, CT, MRI, and digital microscopy complement laboratory findings in parasitic disease detection.
- *Learn Quality Assurance and Biosafety Principles*: Appreciate the importance of laboratory quality control, biosafety protocols, and standard operating procedures (SOPs) in maintaining diagnostic accuracy.
- *Explore Diagnostic Algorithms and Interpretation*: Apply stepwise diagnostic algorithms for common parasitic infections and interpret laboratory findings effectively.
- *Embrace Advances in Point-of-care and Molecular Technologies*: Discover emerging diagnostic innovations, such as AI-assisted microscopy, multiplex assays, and lab-on-a-chip devices, shaping the future of parasitology.
- *Acknowledge Limitations and Pitfalls*: Understand common diagnostic errors, false results, and the need for clinical correlation to improve reliability.

9.1 BASIC DIAGNOSTIC TECHNIQUES IN PARASITOLOGY

Diagnosing parasitic infections requires a multifaceted approach that combines epidemiological information, clinical symptoms, and laboratory testing. Microscopy remains the cornerstone of parasitological diagnostics, especially in field and low-resource settings, as it provides a direct visualization of parasites and allows for epidemiological assessment of parasite burden. However, molecular techniques such as polymerase chain reaction (PCR), real-time PCR, loop-mediated isothermal amplification (LAMP), and Luminex xMAP are increasingly being used to enhance the sensitivity and specificity of parasite identification. Immunological assays like enzyme immunoassays and immunoblotting also play a significant role in the diagnosis of parasitic diseases. The selection of appropriate examination methods and specimen collection sites is crucial for accurate diagnosis, as different approaches show varying sensitivity and specificity to different parasite species and life stages. This chapter will provide an overview of the current and emerging diagnostic techniques for parasitic infections, their advantages, limitations, and applicability in endemic and non-endemic settings.

9.2 SPECIMENS FOR DIAGNOSIS

The examination of different specimens is a crucial step in diagnosing parasitic infections. Various specimens are collected and examined for the presence of parasites, each requiring specific diagnostic approaches. Specimens that are commonly used to diagnose parasitic infections include stool, urine, sputum, blood, and urogenital swab.

Other specimens that can be used include liver aspirates, duodenal aspirates, bile, corneal scrapings, contact lens fluid, cerebrospinal fluid (CSF), tissue samples, including biopsies, and nasal discharge. For instance, stool is examined for the detection of intestinal parasites such as *Giardia lamblia* and *Cryptosporidium parvum* using microscopy and molecular techniques like PCR. Urine, sputum, liver aspirates, duodenal aspirates, bile, corneal scrapings, and contact lens fluid are also examined for parasites like *Schistosoma* and *Paragonimus* using microscopy and serology. Blood is examined for parasites like *Plasmodium* using thin and thick films, while cerebrospinal fluid (CSF) is examined for parasites like *Toxoplasma gondii* using microscopy and PCR. Tissue samples, including biopsies and surgical specimens, are examined for parasites like *Echinococcus* and *Taenia* using histopathology and molecular techniques. These specimens are collected and transported according to specific guidelines to ensure the integrity of the parasites and the accuracy of the diagnostic tests.

9.3 SPECIMEN COLLECTION, HANDLING, AND EXAMINATION

Laboratory diagnosis of parasites is mainly based on the gross examination of the specimen and viewing it under the microscope. The culture of parasites is not routinely done. Methods for detecting parasites in various specimens include:

- **Microscopy**
- **Molecular techniques** such as PCR, LAMP, and Luminex Xmap
- **Immunological/serological assays** such as enzyme immunoassays and immunoblotting (Western blot)

Other methods of diagnosis include imaging tests such as X-rays, ultrasounds, and CT scans.

9.4 MICROSCOPY

Microscopy remains a cornerstone of diagnostic methods for detecting parasitic infections. It involves the direct visualization of parasites and their various life stages through microscopic examination of different clinical specimens. The diagnosis of intestinal parasites typically relies on the microscopic detection of egg, larval, trophozoite, cyst, and/or oocyst life stages in human stool samples.

9.4.1 SPECIMEN COLLECTION AND PREPARATION

Specimens such as blood, stool, urine, sputum, cerebrospinal fluid, aspirates, and biopsies constitute the primary materials collected for the microscopic examination of parasitic infections. The accurate diagnosis of these infections critically depends on meticulous specimen collection, proper transport, and precise processing techniques to preserve parasite integrity. To facilitate optimal visualization and identification under the microscope, various staining methods – including Giemsa, Wright, and modified acid-fast stains – are employed. These stains enhance the morphological features of parasites, enabling differentiation of species and life stages. Adherence to stringent protocols for specimen handling ensures the reliability of laboratory results and supports effective clinical decision-making in parasitology.

9.4.2 STOOL SPECIMEN

A stool specimen is the primary specimen examined at the laboratory for parasites. The results for the specimen rely on the quality and freshness of the stool submitted. Trophozoite stages of parasites are only found in fresh stool because they cannot survive outside the host environment for long periods of time. Fresh stool specimens are therefore examined within 30 minutes of passage for liquid specimens and within one hour for soft specimens.

A gross examination of the faecal specimen to determine its consistency, presence of blood or mucus, and any visible signs of worms or proglottids before any microscopic analysis is done.

Stool submitted to the laboratory is in three consistencies: **Formed, semi-formed, and loose or watery.** The consistency of the stool determines the stage of the parasitic infection.

Concentrating the stool specimen by sedimentation or flotation can increase the sensitivity of detection, especially for small numbers of parasites. Although this method may destroy trophozoites, it enhances the detection of cysts, helminth eggs, and larvae

Stool specimens undergo macroscopic examination to identify the presence of blood, mucus, and proglottids and worms. Microscopic examination involves identifying cysts, trophozoites.

9.4.2.1 Stool Sample Collection

It is recommended that three separate stool specimens be collected on three separate days, ideally in the morning, to ensure detection of intestinal parasites.

The stool specimen collected should not be contaminated with water, as it may tamper with the results. Stool samples should be preserved in 10% formalin if the sample will not be observed immediately. Stool samples that will be observed immediately are then prepared for microscopic examination.

9.4.3 PREPARATION FOR MICROSCOPIC EXAMINATION

For microscopic examination of stool samples, there are a few common preparation methods:

9.4.3.1 Direct Wet Mount Technique

The direct wet mount technique serves as a fundamental diagnostic tool in parasitological stool examination. It involves placing a small amount of fresh stool on a microscope slide, mixing it with a drop of physiological saline or iodine, and covering it with a coverslip for microscopic observation. This method enables the rapid detection of motile protozoan trophozoites, cysts, ova, and larvae. Its simplicity and speed make it especially valuable in preliminary screening and resource-limited settings. However, the technique has a relatively low sensitivity compared to concentration methods, which makes it insufficient as a sole diagnostic approach. Therefore, it is typically used alongside other methods to improve detection accuracy. The direct wet mount's effectiveness depends greatly on specimen freshness and prompt examination, as protozoan trophozoites deteriorate quickly outside the host.

- ***Saline wet mount***

  The saline mount technique is used to demonstrate the morphology of parasites in stool specimens. They are particularly preferred for observing motile trophozoites of parasites like *Giardia lamblia*.

  The technique involves mixing a small amount of stool with physiological saline to create a wet mount, which is then examined under a microscope.

  Methodology:
  - Fresh stool samples are used for the preparation of the wet mount.
  - A small amount of stool is mixed with physiological saline to create a uniform emulsion.
  - A drop of the emulsion is then placed on a microscope slide and a coverslip is gently placed over it to spread out the emulsion into a thin transparent layer.
- ***Iodine wet mount***

  The iodine mount technique is commonly used to differentiate and identify parasites based on their morphological features and internal structures. Iodine stains the glycogen masses of protozoan cysts, making them more visible. Iodine kills trophozoites, facilitating the visualization of parasitic ova and cyst morphology.

  Methodology:

  For iodine mounts: The iodine mount can also be preserved for longer if the coverslip is sealed with paraffin oil or petroleum jelly.
  - A small amount of stool is placed on a microscope slide.
  - A drop of iodine solution (usually 1% iodine) is added.
  - The slide is covered with a coverslip.
  - The preparation is examined under a microscope
- ***Methylene blue-glycerol mount technique***

  The methylene blue-glycerol mount technique is used to enhance the visualization of parasitic morphology and internal structures in stool specimens, especially for medically important intestinal parasites. It involves combining methylene blue dye with glycerol to create a wet mount that provides better contrast and clarity for microscopic observation.
  - Fresh stool samples are used for the preparation of the wet mount.
  - Methylene blue dye is added to the faecal sample to stain the parasites.

- Glycerol is added to the stained sample to create a wet mount.
- The preparation is examined under the microscope to visualize the morphology and internal structures of parasites.

- ***Iron haematoxylin technique***

  The iron haematoxylin technique is a traditional staining method used for the detection and identification of intestinal protozoa. The stain is made up of a combination of haematoxylin, haematin, and oxyhaematin. Haematin acts as the mordant to produce a lake, which reacts with ferric ammonium sulphate to form the ferric lake (iron haematoxylin), a basic dye.

  Reagents to be used include:

  - ***Schaudinn's fixative***: Mercuric chloride, ethanol, acetic acid
  - ***Iodine solution***: Ethanol, tincture of iodine
  - ***Mordant-differentiating solution***: Iron alum (ferric ammonium sulphate), hydrochloric acid
  - ***Haematoxylin solution***: Haematoxylin in distilled water

  Fixation in Schaudinn's solution preserves the morphology of the parasite while iron haematoxylin binds to nucleic acids. Acid alcohol removes excess stain.

  Methodology:

  - For fresh stool samples, prepare a thin smear on a slide and air dry. For preserved samples (PVA or SAF-fixed), mix the sample, transfer to a paper towel, apply to a slide, and air dry completely.
  - Fix the dried smear in Schaudinn's solution for 30 minutes. Rinse in 70% ethanol.
  - Stain in iron haematoxylin solution for 5–10 minutes.
  - Rinse briefly in tap water.
  - Differentiate in 1% acid alcohol for 5–10 seconds.
  - Rinse in tap water until nuclei turn blue (2 minutes).
  - Dehydrate through graded ethanol (70%, 80%, 95%, and 100%).
  - Clear in xylene.
  - Mount with a permanent medium.

- ***The Wheatley's trichrome technique***

  The Wheatley's trichrome technique involves staining stool or faecal film samples with a combination of dyes to facilitate the detection and identification of intestinal protozoa. The stain contains two dyes: Chromotrope 2R and Light Green SF. Chromotrope 2R stains nuclear chromatin, chromatid bodies, karyosomes, parasite eggs and larvae, bacteria, and ingested erythrocytes red to purple-red. Light Green SF stains the cytoplasm of preserved cysts, trophozoites, and cellular constituents blue-green.

Wet mount techniques are not always able to reveal the presence of parasites. This is due to the fact that the parasite count may be too small. Concentration techniques can help improve the visibility of parasites in stool.

9.4.4 CONCENTRATION TECHNIQUES

Concentration techniques increase the ability to detect protozoan cysts, helminth eggs, and larvae by reducing the amount of artefacts in the stool sample. These techniques are done after direct examination with the wet mount techniques as trophozoites are not found in concentrated samples. Two methods are generally employed for routine use in the laboratory: Sedimentation and flotation methods.

9.4.4.1 Sedimentation Method

The sedimentation method involves stool suspension in fluids with lower specific gravity than the parasite cysts, eggs, or larvae such as water, physiological saline, or ether which enable the parasitic forms to sediment. The sedimentation method is particularly used to concentrate protozoan cysts, helminth eggs, and larvae. It is the easiest routine method to perform and is subject to the least technical error. The sedimentation method can be done by two ways; the simple method by gravity and the formalin-ether centrifugal sedimentation method.

9.4.4.2 General Sedimentation Methodology

- About 2 mL of fresh stool sample is added to a penicillin bottle containing 10 mL of saline or 10% formaldehyde and shaken to form a uniform suspension.
- The suspension is transferred to a 15 mL test tube or left to stand for about one hour or centrifuged for 3 minutes at 1,800 rpm.
- The supernatant is discarded.
- The suspension is then resuspended in water and made to stand for one hour or recentrifuged at 1800 rpm for 3

minutes. This process is repeated until the supernatant is relatively clear.

- The sediment is then mixed with formalin and ether.
- A bit of the sediment is then removed with a Pasteur pipette, and a wet mount is prepared.

9.4.5 FLOTATION METHOD

In the flotation method, the parasites are suspended in fluids that have a higher specific gravity than the parasite to be observed, such as a saturated solution of sodium chloride. This method is preferred to view the presence of hookworms, roundworms, tapeworms, and whipworms. It cannot be used to concentrate protozoan cysts, as harsh chemical solutions can distort the cysts.

9.4.5.1 General Floatation Methodology

- A small amount of the stool sample is transferred to a penicillin bottle containing the Willis solution.
- The bottle is filled to the top and a coverslip is carefully placed on the top of the suspension without introducing air bubbles.
- After about 10 minutes, the coverslip is taken out, mounted on a slide and viewed promptly.

9.4.6 URINE SPECIMEN

Urine is usually tested for the presence of blood fluke infections such as schistosomiasis caused by *Schistosoma haematobium*. It can also be used to detect parasites such as *Trichomonas vaginalis*. The urine is usually collected around 10 am to 2 pm, when the parasites are more active, and after the patient has been made to undergo physical exercise such as running. This enables the dislodging of parasites from the walls of the bladder. Urinalysis can also be used to detect any abnormalities in the urine caused by parasitic organisms.

Before observing urine under the microscope, the urine is first observed macroscopically. Macroscopic examination of the urine involves the visual observation of the physical characteristics of the urine sample, such as colour, turbidity, and odour, the presence of foam or bubbles, and concentration.

Wet mount is the best technique for observing urine under the microscope. It involves placing a drop of urine sediment on a slide and examining it under a microscope.

Staining the drop of urine with dyes like methylene blue or eosin can help visualize parasites and their internal structures in more detail.

9.4.6.1 Blood Specimen

Microscopic examination of Giemsa-stained thick and thin blood smears is the standard procedure for detecting blood parasites like those that cause malaria, trypanosomiasis, and lymphatic filariasis.

Blood smears are prepared from capillary blood from the finger or venous blood collected in EDTA tubes. Blood smears should be prepared within 3 hours of blood collection and stained with either 10% or 20% diluted Giemsa stain for about ten to thirty minutes.

9.4.6.1.1 THICK BLOOD FILM PREPARATION

- Collect venous blood sample in an EDTA anticoagulant tube or capillary blood from the finger.
- Place two large drops (approximately 10–20 μL each) of well-mixed blood onto the centre of a clean glass slide.
- Spread the blood drops rapidly and evenly across the slide using the corner of another slide, creating a thick, circular smear about 1 cm in diameter.
- Allow the thick film to air dry completely, without fixing.

9.4.6.1.2 THIN BLOOD FILM PREPARATION

- Place a small drop (2–3 μL) of well-mixed venous blood near one end of a clean glass slide.
- Using a second slide held at a 30–45° angle, quickly spread the blood drop into a thin, feathered smear across the slide.
- Allow the thin film to air dry completely.
- Fix the thin film by dipping it briefly (2–3 seconds) in methanol.

9.4.6.1.3 NB

- The thick film allows concentration of parasites for detection, while the thin film enables identification of parasite species.
- Thick films should not be fixed, as this interferes with haemolysis and parasite visualization.
- Thin films must be fixed with methanol to preserve cell morphology.
- Proper drying and staining (e.g., Giemsa) of both thick and thin films is crucial for effective microscopic examination.
- Systematic viewing of the stained films under oil immersion is required to detect and identify any blood parasites present.
- The lab technician identifies the parasites, such as filarial worms and trypanosomes, based on their morphology, such as shape, size, and staining characteristics.
- The lab technician estimates the number of parasites present in the blood sample by counting the number of parasitized red blood cells (RBCs) per 10,000 RBCs. This is done by examining a well-stained thin blood film.
- The lab technician reports the results, including the type and number of parasites present, as well as any other relevant information.

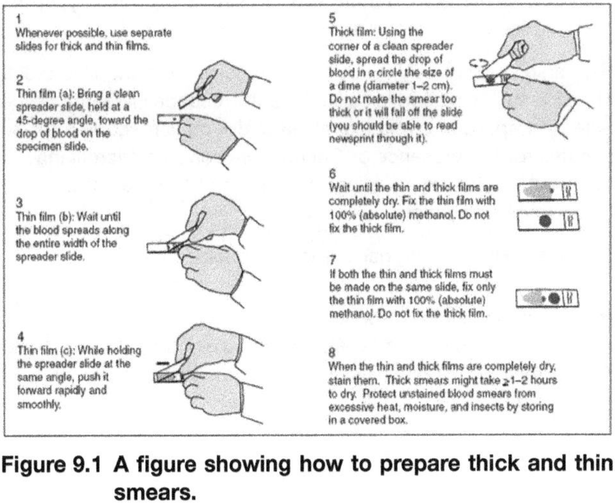

Figure 9.1 A figure showing how to prepare thick and thin smears.

9.4.7 SPUTUM SPECIMEN

This type of specimen is submitted to the lab for diagnosis of parasites that invade the respiratory system, such as *Ascaris lumbricoides*. Laboratory examination for parasites from this sample type is uncertain because parasites are rarely coughed up.

9.4.8 SKIN SPECIMEN

Skin snips and skin scrapings are important diagnostic techniques used to detect parasitic infections in humans. These minimally invasive procedures involve collecting samples from the skin and examining them under a microscope to identify the presence of parasites such as *Sarcoptes scabiei*, *Loa loa*, and *Onchocerca volvulus*.

Proper handling and processing of skin samples are crucial for accurate diagnosis. Factors like fixation, dehydration, clearing, infiltration, and embedding can all impact the preservation and visualization of parasites in the samples. Additionally, expertise is required to correctly identify the parasites present under the microscope, as many species can appear similar at certain life stages.

9.4.9 SKIN SNIPS

Skin snip is the gold standard for detecting and identifying the microfilariae of *Onchocerca volvulus*.

Skin snip involves taking a snip of the skin from the iliac crest. The skin snip is placed in saline on a microscope slide, the tissue is teased apart, and it is examined under a microscope after 30 minutes for the presence of *Onchocerca volvulus* microfilariae. If the initial results are negative, the sample should be left to stand for up to 4 hours before re-examining.

However, skin snipping has some drawbacks:

- It can be painful for patients.
- There's a potential risk of transmitting blood-borne infections.
- It may not be sensitive enough to detect early or mild infections.

9.4.9.1 Skin Snipping Procedure

- Apply topical anaesthetic cream to the areas where snips will be taken.
- Collect eight skin snips from several sites, usually over bony prominences like the shoulder, buttocks, external thigh, and calves. Additional snips may be taken from itchy areas.
- Each snip should be about 2 × 1 mm in size.
- Use forceps to lift the skin slightly and cut the small piece with a sterile scalpel or punch biopsy tool.
- Place each skin snip immediately in saline solution on a labelled glass slide.
- Tease apart the tissue on the slide.
- Cover the sample with a coverslip.
- Examine under a microscope after 30 minutes for the presence of *Onchocerca volvulus* microfilariae.
- If results are initially negative, let the sample stand for up to 4 hours before re-examining.

9.4.10 SKIN SCRAPINGS

Skin scrapings are used to diagnose various parasitic skin infections, particularly mite infestations like scabies.

Skin scraping involves scraping the superficial layer of the skin with a blunt instrument, such as a disposable lancet.

The collected material is then examined under a microscope to look for parasites, eggs, or faecal pellets.

To enhance the sensitivity of parasite detection in skin samples, various concentration techniques such as centrifugation, filtration and sedimentation can be used.

9.4.10.1 Skin Scraping Procedure

- Place a large drop of mineral oil in the centre of the labelled slide.
- Locate an area of alopecia, scale, crusts, hyperpigmentation, papules, or erythema. Apply a few drops of mineral oil to the skin area to be sampled. This helps trap the material for collection.
- Apply slight pressure to the skin surface to keep it from bunching up.

- Hold the flat portion of the blade at a right angle to the skin surface. Advance the blade in the same direction as the hair growth, using broad strokes to collect a sample from a large area while holding the skin taut. Scrape large areas and multiple areas to maximize sample collection.
- Collect the sample of scale, crusts, epithelial cells, and keratin debris in the mineral oil on the blade by using an upward scooping motion.
- For suspected *Sarcoptes scabiei*, perform at least 5–10 scrapes, targeting areas like the ear pinna margins, elbows, hocks, papular regions, or areas with excessive crusts and scales.
- Transfer the collected material from the blade to the slide with mineral oil.
- Gently lower a coverslip over the sample, avoiding air bubbles.
- Examine the slide under a microscope at 10× and 40× magnification, scanning multiple fields to look for parasites, eggs, or faecal material.

9.4.11 BIOPSY SPECIMEN

Diagnosing parasitic infections from biopsies involves a series of steps to ensure accurate identification of the parasite. This procedure is crucial for confirming infections, especially when non-invasive methods are inconclusive. The procedure to detect parasites in biopsies involves:

- ***Sample collection***: The appropriate biopsy site is selected based on the suspected parasite. For example, intestinal biopsies are suitable for *Giardia lamblia*, while muscle biopsies are preferred for *Trichinella* spp. An adequate tissue sample is collected, ensuring it includes both affected and adjacent normal tissue for comparison.
- ***Fixation***: Immediately fix the tissue sample in 10% buffered formalin to preserve cellular and tissue architecture. For molecular studies, a portion of the sample can be preserved in RNA later® Solution or frozen at −80°C.
- ***Embedding***: Embed the fixed tissue in paraffin wax to facilitate sectioning.
- ***Sectioning and staining***: Thin sections (3–5 µm) of the paraffin-embedded tissue are cut using a microtome. Stain the sections with Haematoxylin and Eosin (H&E) for general histopathological examination. Special stains like Giemsa,

Trichrome, or Periodic Acid-Schiff (PAS) can be used to highlight specific parasites or structures.

- ***Microscopic examination***: The stained sections are examined under a light microscope while looking for characteristic features of the parasite, such as trophozoites, cysts, or larvae.
- ***Immunohistochemistry***: Use parasite-specific antibodies to stain the tissue sections. This method enhances the visibility of parasites that may be difficult to detect with routine stains.
- ***Digestion method (for muscle biopsies)***: Muscle tissue is digested in a solution of pepsin and hydrochloric acid to break down muscle fibres and release encysted larvae. Filter the digestate and examine it under a microscope to identify free larvae.

When microscopy does not yield adequate results, molecular techniques and serological assays are used to detect parasites from various types of samples.

Culturing of parasites is ideally not practised because it is very difficult to grow parasitic organisms in the lab.

9.4.12 IMPORTANCE OF TIMING, FIXATIVES, AND STORAGE CONDITIONS

When dealing with parasitic organisms, proper collection, preservation, and storage techniques are crucial for accurate identification, morphological studies, and downstream molecular analyses.

9.4.12.1 Timing

- Ideally, parasites should be collected alive or freshly killed to ensure optimal morphology and minimize degradation.
- Delays in fixation can cause internal organ degeneration, autolysis (self-digestion of tissues), and loss of delicate structures.
- External parasites like mites or fleas can be collected directly from the host or preserved in vials with 10% formaldehyde.
- Internal parasites require careful dissection from the host tissue to minimize damage.
- For some parasites, targeting specific life stages is crucial. Encysted stages or eggs may require different protocols than adult worms.

9.4.12.2 Fixatives

- Fixatives preserve the parasite's three-dimensional structure and prevent decay.
- The choice of fixative depends on the intended purpose of the study.
- Common fixatives for parasites include:
  - ***Formalin (10% neutral buffered formalin)***: A widely used general fixative that preserves overall morphology.
  - ***Alcohol (70% ethanol)***: Suitable for mites, fleas, and other external parasites. It is a good choice for short-term preservation.
  - ***Glutaraldehyde***: Excellent for preserving ultrastructure for electron microscopy studies.
  - ***Alcohol-formalin-acetic acid (AFA)***: Effective for preserving both morphology and DNA for molecular analyses.

9.4.12.3 Storage Conditions

- Properly fixed parasites can be stored for long periods.
- Specimens should be kept in airtight containers submerged in the chosen fixative.
- Labelling the container with parasite identification, collection date, and fixative type is essential for proper record keeping.
- For long-term storage, refrigeration (4°C) is recommended to slow down any enzymatic activity that could degrade the parasite.
- Freezing (–20°C or colder) is suitable for some parasites intended for molecular studies.

9.5 MOLECULAR TECHNIQUES

9.5.1 POLYMERASE CHAIN REACTION (PCR)

PCR-based methods are powerful tools for the diagnosis of parasitic infections. Studies have demonstrated the successful application of PCR techniques for the detection and quantification of protozoan parasites like *Plasmodium* spp., *Cryptosporidium* spp., and *Entamoeba* spp., as well as helminth parasites such as *Schistosoma* spp. and soil-transmitted helminths. While PCR-based methods require specialized equipment and expertise, they are increasingly being integrated into routine clinical diagnostics for parasitic diseases, complementing traditional microscopy

- Compared to traditional microscopy, PCR offers several key advantages:
  - Higher sensitivity and specificity in detecting parasite DNA, allowing diagnosis even at low parasite densities.
  - Ability to identify and quantify different parasite species, including in mixed infections.
  - Potential for detecting genetic markers associated with drug resistance.
  - Suitability for use with a variety of sample types, including blood, stool, and environmental samples.

PCR involves three main steps that are repeated in cycles to exponentially amplify a target DNA sequence:

Denaturation: The DNA sample is heated to 94–98°C to separate the double-stranded DNA into single strands.

Annealing: The temperature is lowered to allow short DNA sequences called primers to bind to complementary sequences flanking the target region on the single-stranded DNA.

Extension: DNA polymerase, typically Taq polymerase, synthesizes new DNA strands complementary to the template DNA, using the primers as starting points.

These three steps are repeated for 20–40 cycles, with each cycle doubling the amount of target DNA. The primers are designed to be specific to the target sequence, allowing selective amplification.

Key components of a PCR reaction include:

- DNA template containing the target sequence
- DNA polymerase (e.g., Taq polymerase)
- Primers complementary to the target region
- Deoxynucleotides (dNTPs) as building blocks
- Buffer solution providing optimal conditions

Variations of standard PCR include:

- Real-time PCR for quantification
- Nested PCR for improved specificity
- Multiplex PCR for amplifying multiple targets simultaneously
- Reverse transcription PCR (RT-PCR) for amplifying RNA targets

To obtain a DNA sample from a parasite before performing PCR:

- Collect the appropriate sample type containing the parasite, such as blood, stool, or tissue. For example, collect a stool sample for intestinal parasites or a blood sample for blood-borne parasites like *Plasmodium*.
- Preserve the sample in a fixative or preservative compatible with molecular detection, such as TotalFix, Unifix, modified PVA, or Ecofix. This allows storage and shipping at room temperature. Alternatively, store unpreserved samples at 4°C or frozen with dry ice.
- Extract the parasite DNA from the sample using a DNA extraction kit or protocol optimized for the parasite and sample type. Common methods include the FastDNA kit, phenol-chloroform extraction, or commercial kits like the QIAamp DNA Mini Kit.
- Mechanical or chemical lysis may be required to break open the parasite cells and release the DNA, especially for hardy parasites like helminths. Techniques include bead-beating, freeze-thaw cycles, or enzymatic digestion.
- Purify the extracted DNA to remove PCR inhibitors that may be present in the sample, such as heme compounds in blood or polysaccharides in stool. Spin column purification kits are commonly used for this purpose.
- Quantify and assess the quality of the purified DNA using spectrophotometry or gel electrophoresis to ensure sufficient quantity and purity for PCR amplification.
- Store the extracted DNA at 4°C for short-term use or –20°C/–80°C for long-term storage until ready to perform PCR.

9.5.2 LOOP-MEDIATED ISOTHERMAL AMPLIFICATION (LAMP)

LAMP has emerged as a powerful molecular technique for the rapid and accurate detection of various parasitic infections. LAMP is a rapid, sensitive, and specific nucleic acid amplification technique that can be performed under isothermal conditions, typically between 60°C and 65°C, without the need for thermal cycling equipment required for PCR.

Compared to traditional microscopy and PCR methods, LAMP offers several key advantages:

- ***High sensitivity and specificity***: LAMP can detect parasite DNA at very low levels, with sensitivity often exceeding that of PCR.
- ***Rapid and simple procedure***: LAMP can be performed in under an hour, without the need for expensive thermal cyclers required for PCR.
- ***Colourimetric readout***: Many LAMP assays utilize a colour change readout, allowing visual detection of positive results, making them suitable for resource-limited settings.

LAMP has been successfully applied for the detection of a wide range of parasitic infections, including Malaria (*Plasmodium* spp.), Leishmaniasis (*Leishmania* spp.), Chagas disease (*Trypanosoma cruzi*), Schistosomiasis (*Schistosoma* spp.), Filariasis (*Onchocerca, Loa, Mansonella*), intestinal parasites (*Giardia lamblia, Cryptosporidium parvum, Entamoeba histolytica*).

The key steps in the LAMP methodology are:

- ***Primer design***: LAMP utilizes a set of 4–6 specially designed primers that recognize 6–8 distinct regions on the target DNA sequence. This includes two inner primers (FIP and BIP), two outer primers (F3 and B3), and optionally two loop primers (LF and LB) to accelerate the reaction.
- ***Isothermal amplification***: The reaction mixture containing the sample DNA, primers, DNA polymerase (e.g., Bst polymerase), dNTPs, and buffer is incubated at a constant temperature. The polymerase initiates DNA synthesis using the inner primers, while the outer primers help displace the newly synthesized strands.
- ***Strand displacement***: The DNA synthesis and strand displacement create loop structures that serve as templates for further amplification. This cyclic amplification leads to the rapid and exponential accumulation of target DNA.
- ***Detection***: LAMP amplification can be detected using various methods, such as:
    - ***Visual colour change***: Addition of a pH-sensitive dye like phenol red or calcein allows visual detection of a positive reaction by a colour change.
    - ***Turbidity***: The large amount of amplified DNA products causes turbidity that can be measured by a turbidimeter.
    - ***Fluorescence***: Intercalating fluorescent dyes like SYBR Green can be used to monitor the reaction in real time.

9.6 SEROLOGICAL TESTS

Serological tests constitute a pivotal component in the diagnostic arsenal of parasitology. These tests are in vitro assays designed to detect specific antibodies produced by the host in response to parasitic infections or, alternatively, to identify parasite-derived antigens circulating in the host's body fluids. By focusing on the immune response rather than directly detecting the parasite, serological assays can reveal evidence of infection even when parasites are present in low numbers or difficult to visualize microscopically.

The primary advantage of serological testing lies in its ability to aid diagnosis in cases where direct parasitological methods fall short, such as occult infections or chronic stages where parasite load is minimal. Serological tests encompass a wide variety of methodologies, including ELISA, immunofluorescence assays (IFA), agglutination tests, and Western blotting, among others. These techniques exploit the specificity of antigen–antibody reactions to enable sensitive and, where applicable, quantitative detection.

While serology offers substantial benefits, including epidemiological surveillance and monitoring of treatment efficacy, interpretation necessitates consideration of antibody persistence, cross-reactivity among related parasites, and the clinical context.

9.6.1 ENZYME IMMUNOASSAYS

Enzyme immunoassays (EIAs), such as ELISA, are widely used for the serodiagnosis of parasitic infections due to their sensitivity and ease of performance.

Key advantages of EIAs include:

- Ability to test large numbers of samples
- Quantitative results
- Potential for automation

EIAs leverage the specific binding between an antigen and its corresponding antibody. An enzyme-labelled antibody is used to detect the presence of the target antigen in a sample. The enzyme catalyses a reaction that produces a measurable signal (colour change or fluorescence) proportional to the amount of antigen present. EIAs have been successfully applied for the diagnosis of infections like trichinellosis, hydatidosis, schistosomiasis, toxoplasmosis, African trypanosomiasis, and amoebiasis. They can detect specific antibody classes (IgG, IgM, and IgA) to aid in determining the stage of infection.

9.6.2 *IMMUNOBLOTTING*

Immunoblotting, also known as Western blot, is a confirmatory test that uses electrophoretically separated parasite antigens to detect specific antibodies in patients. It offers high specificity by identifying antibodies against multiple antigenic components of the parasite. Immunoblotting is often used as a supplementary test to resolve indeterminate or false-positive EIA results. It has been employed for diagnosing infections such as Chagas disease, cysticercosis, and toxoplasmosis. While EIAs are suitable for large-scale screening, immunoblotting provides a more definitive diagnosis, especially in cases of cross-reactivity with other pathogens. The combination of sensitive EIA screening followed by specific immunoblot confirmation is a powerful approach for accurate serological diagnosis of parasitic infections.

The technique offers high specificity, but may require more expertise and resources compared to simpler serological assays like ELISA.

9.7 IMAGING TESTS

Imaging tests, such as X-rays, ultrasounds, and CT scans, can be used to detect cystic lesions and calcifications caused by parasitic worms such as *Taenia* spp. A mass of worms can also be detected by imaging tests.

9.7.1 *X-RAYS*

- Use electromagnetic radiation to create 2D images of dense structures like bones and some organs.
- Best for visualizing bone fractures, lung conditions, and some dental issues.
- Quick and inexpensive, but provide limited soft tissue detail.
- Involve a small amount of radiation exposure.

9.7.2 ULTRASOUND

- Uses high-frequency sound waves to create real-time images of soft tissues and organs.
- Excellent for visualizing soft tissues, blood flow, and moving structures.
- Commonly used for pregnancy, abdominal organs, and cardiovascular imaging.
- No radiation exposure, safe for repeated use.
- Limited effectiveness in imaging structures behind bone or air.

9.7.3 COMPUTED TOMOGRAPHY (CT) SCANS

- Combine multiple X-ray images taken from different angles to create detailed 3D images.
- Provide excellent detail of both soft tissues and bones.
- Useful for diagnosing a wide range of conditions, including tumours, internal injuries, and vascular diseases.
- Higher radiation exposure compared to standard X-rays.
- It can show more detail than X-rays or ultrasound for many conditions.

9.8 CURRENT ADVANCES IN DIAGNOSTICS

The field of parasitology has witnessed remarkable progress in diagnostic technology, driven by innovations in molecular biology, immunology, and digital science. These advances have greatly improved the accuracy, speed, and accessibility of parasite detection and identification.

9.8.1 DIGITAL AND AUTOMATED MICROSCOPY

Artificial Intelligence (AI) and Machine Learning: AI-powered digital microscopes can automatically detect and classify parasites in blood smears or stool samples, reducing human error and increasing throughput, especially in resource-limited settings.

9.8.2 MULTIPLEX AND SYNDROMIC PANELS

Modern diagnostic platforms can now simultaneously detect multiple pathogens – including parasites, bacteria, and viruses – from a single sample. This approach is especially valuable in cases of undifferentiated febrile or gastrointestinal illnesses.

9.8.3 PORTABLE AND FIELD-DEPLOYABLE DEVICES

Biosensors and Lab-on-a-Chip Technologies: Miniaturized devices are being developed to integrate sample processing and detection, allowing for rapid, on-site diagnosis of parasitic infections in remote or resource-limited areas.

9.8.4 PROTEOMICS AND METABOLOMICS

Large-scale analysis of parasite proteins and metabolites is leading to the discovery of novel biomarkers, which may enable earlier diagnosis and improved differentiation between parasite species

9.9 DEFINITIONS

Morphology *refers to observing the size, shape, and physical features of parasites to help identify what kind they are.*

Giemsa stain *is a special dye used in laboratories to colour cells and parasites, making them easier to see under a microscope*

EDTA *stands for ethylenediaminetetraacetic acid. It is a chemical used in medical laboratories as an anticoagulant to prevent blood from clotting during collection and testing.*

Haemolysis *is the process where red blood cells break open and release their contents, including haemoglobin, into the surrounding fluid such as blood plasma.*

FURTHER READING

Darwish, I. A. (2006). Immunoassay methods and their applications in pharmaceutical analysis: Basic methodology and recent advances. *International Journal of Biomedical Science: IJBS*, 2(3), 217–235.

Kandi, V. (2017). Laboratory diagnosis of scabies using a simple saline mount: A clinical microbiologist's report. *Cureus*, 9(3), e1102. https://doi.org/10.7759/cureus.1102

Kashir, J., & Yaqinuddin, A. (2020). Loop mediated isothermal amplification (LAMP) assays as a rapid diagnostic for COVID-19. *Medical Hypotheses*, 141, 109786. https://doi.org/10.1016/j.mehy.2020.109786

Kasirga, E. (2019). The importance of stool tests in diagnosis and follow-up of gastrointestinal disorders in children. *Turkish Archives of Pediatrics/Türk Pediatri Arşivi*, 54(3), 141–148. https://doi.org/10.14744/TurkPediatriArs.2018.00483

Khanna, V., Tilak, K., Rasheed, S., & Mukhopadhyay, C. (2014). Identification and preservation of intestinal parasites using methylene blue-glycerol mount: A new approach to stool microscopy. *Journal of Parasitology Research*, 672018, 4 pages. https://doi.org/10.1155/2014/672018

Lou, J., Yu, Y., & Dai, F. (2016). Laboratory test for diagnosis of parasitic diseases. *Radiology of Parasitic Diseases: A Practical Approach*, 25–46. https://doi.org/10.1007/978-94-024-0911-6_6

Mahittikorn, A., Masangkay, F. R., Kotepui, K. U., et al. (2021). Comparative performance of PCR using DNA extracted from dried blood spots and whole blood samples for malaria diagnosis: A meta-analysis. *Scientific Reports*, 11, 4845. https://doi.org/10.1038/s41598-021-83977-5

Meurs, L., Polderman, A. M., S. Vinkeles Melchers, N. V., T. Brienen, E. A., Verweij, J. J., Groosjohan, B., Mendes, F., Mechendura, M., Hepp, D. H., C. Langenberg, M. C., Edelenbosch, R., & Polman, K. (2017). Diagnosing polyparasitism in a high-prevalence setting in Beira, Mozambique: Detection of intestinal parasites in fecal samples by microscopy and real-time PCR. *PLoS Neglected Tropical Diseases*, 11(1), e0005310. https://doi.org/10.1371/journal.pntd.0005310

Momčilović, S., Cantacessi, C., Arsić-Arsenijević, V., Otranto, D., & Tasić-Otašević, S. (2019). Rapid diagnosis of parasitic diseases: Current scenario and future needs. *Clinical Microbiology and Infection*, 25(3), 290–309. https://doi.org/10.1016/j.cmi.2018.04.028

Oberhuber, G., Mesteri, I., Kopf, W., & Müller, H. (2016). Demonstration of Trophozoites of G. Lamblia in ileal mucosal biopsy specimens may reveal giardiasis in patients with significantly inflamed parasite-free duodenal mucosa. *The American Journal of Surgical Pathology*, 40(9), 1280–1285. https://doi.org/10.1097/PAS.0000000000000665

Porstmann, T., & Kiessig, S. T. (1992). Enzyme immunoassay techniques. An overview. *Journal of Immunological Methods*, 150(1–2), 5–21. https://doi.org/10.1016/0022-1759(92)90061-w

Reed S. L., & Davis C. E. (2018). Laboratory diagnosis of parasitic infections. In J. Jameson, A. S. Fauci, D. L. Kasper, S. L. Hauser, D. L. Longo, & J. Loscalzo (Eds.), *Harrison's principles of internal medicine*, 20e. McGraw-Hill Education. https://accessmedicine.mhmedical.com/content.aspx?bookid=2129&sectionid=192510558

Ricciardi, A., & Ndao, M. (2015). Diagnosis of parasitic infections: What's going on? *SLAS Discovery*, 20(1), 6–21. https://doi.org/10.1177/1087057114548065

Rodríguez Carnero, P., Hernández Mateo, P., Martín-Garre, S., García Pérez, Á., & Del Campo, L. (2017). Unexpected hosts: imaging parasitic diseases. *Insights into Imaging*, 8(1), 101–125. https://doi.org/10.1007/s13244-016-0525-2

Schumann, G. B., & Greenberg, N. F. (1979). Usefulness of macroscopic urinalysis as a screening procedure. A preliminary report. *American Journal of Clinical Pathology*, 71(4), 452–456. https://doi.org/10.1093/ajcp/71.4.452

Srirungruang, S., Mahajindawong, B., Nimitpanya, P., Bunkasem, U., Ayuyoe, P., Nuchprayoon, S., & Sanprasert, V. (2022). Comparative study of DNA extraction methods for the PCR detection of intestinal parasites in human stool samples. *Diagnostics* (Basel, Switzerland), 12(11), 2588. https://doi.org/10.3390/diagnostics12112588

10 Pharmacological and Non-pharmacological Management of Parasitic Diseases

The future belongs to those who believe in the beauty of their dreams.

Eleanor Roosevelt

CHAPTER OUTLINE

In this chapter, you will gain a comprehensive understanding of the movement and processing of antiparasitic drugs within the body. Prepare to explore how drugs interact with parasitic infections through the following key topics:

- *Introduction to Pharmacokinetics*: You will be introduced to the concept of pharmacokinetics as the study of drug absorption, distribution, metabolism, and excretion (ADME), highlighting its significance in developing effective treatments against parasitic diseases.
- *Absorption of Antiparasitic Drugs*: You will uncover various modes of drug absorption, including oral, topical, and parenteral routes. Learn about important factors affecting absorption, such as drug properties, pH, food intake, and formulation.
- You will explore mechanisms like passive diffusion, facilitated diffusion, active transport, and pinocytosis that facilitate absorption and understand factors that can enhance or impair this process.
- *Distribution within the Body*: The movement of drugs from the bloodstream to tissues and organs will be examined. Understand how tissue distribution impacts therapeutic and adverse effects, along with important concepts such as plasma protein binding and the pharmacokinetic-pharmacodynamic relationship.
- *Metabolism of Antiparasitic Drugs*: Explore the biochemical processes responsible for drug breakdown primarily in the liver, involving key enzymes like cytochrome P450. You'll see

DOI: 10.1201/9781003733935-10

how metabolism influences drug efficacy and safety, as well as factors such as genetics, age, and drug interactions that can modify metabolism.

- *Excretion of Drugs and Metabolites*: Learn about how drugs and their metabolites are eliminated through renal and biliary routes, and the importance of excretion in treatment effectiveness.
- *Pharmacokinetic Parameters*: Gain knowledge of crucial parameters such as bioavailability, half-life, clearance, and volume of distribution that quantify drug behaviour and guide dosing strategies.
- *Special Considerations in Parasitology*: You will explore unique challenges such as drug penetration into difficult tissues (e.g., crossing the blood–brain barrier), intracellular parasite activity, life cycle stages affecting treatment, and emerging drug resistance.
- *Examples of Key Antiparasitic Drugs*: Study the pharmacokinetics of important drugs like albendazole, ivermectin, and praziquantel, noting their absorption characteristics, metabolism, distribution, and half-lives.
- *Safety and Treatment Implications*: Understand the implications of dosing schedules, drug–drug interactions, and patient-specific factors like age and organ function on therapy safety and effectiveness.
- *Herbal Medicine in Parasitic Disease Treatment*: Discover the historical and ongoing role of herbal remedies in managing parasitic diseases. Learn about common medicinal plants with antiparasitic properties such as neem, garlic, wormwood, thyme, and ginger.
- Explore preparation methods, bioactive compounds, mechanisms of antiparasitic action, and the current scientific evidence supporting herbal efficacy. Consider the challenges in standardization, safety, and regulation of herbal treatments.

10.1 PHARMACOKINETICS OF ANTIPARASITIC DRUGS

Pharmacokinetics refers to the study of the movement of drugs through the body. It describes the study of drug absorption, distribution, metabolism, excretion, and how the body affects the drug and vice versa. To give a broader appreciation of parasitology, pharmacokinetics is crucial for developing effective treatments against parasitic infections. This chapter will explore the key principles of pharmacokinetics in relation to parasitic drugs. Other considerations include bioavailability, absorption rate, factors that can impair absorption and enhance absorption.

As previously mentioned, the pharmacokinetics of antiparasitic drugs follow a process known as ADME (absorption, distribution, metabolism, and excretion).

10.1.1 DRUG ABSORPTION

Absorption is the process by which unmetabolized drugs are transported from the site of administration into the bloodstream, allowing the drug to reach the systemic circulation and its target tissues. This includes the intake of drugs through means such as oral, topical, and parenteral. The factors that affect absorption include physicochemical properties of the drug, pH, food intake, and drug formulation.

- ***Oral absorption***: Most antiparasitic drugs are taken orally.
- ***Topical absorption***: In the case of scabies, drugs like permethrin can be applied to the skin.
- ***Parenteral administration***: Drugs such as antimony compounds for leishmaniasis can be administered intravenously or intramuscularly.

10.1.1.1 Drug Absorption Mechanisms

Various mechanisms are employed to ensure complete absorption. Some of these mechanisms of absorption include:

Passive diffusion: This involves the movement of the drug molecule according to the concentration gradient from a higher drug concentration to a lower concentration until equilibrium is reached.

Facilitated diffusion: This involves a passive movement of molecules along the concentration gradient. As a selective process, it allows only selective molecules and ions to pass through it.

Active transport: This refers to when a substance moves against a concentration gradient.

Pinocytosis: This refers to an active, energy-consuming process where extracellular fluid and solutes are taken up into a cell via small vesicles.

10.1.1.2 Factors that Affect Drug Absorption

For factors that can impair absorption, these include a host of avenues including but not limited to **dietary factors, dose and dosing regimen, formulation factors, and patient factors.**

Dietary factors: This refers to food that a person, animal or community habitually eats. As a hindering factor, it encompasses the high doses of other minerals in the diet, partly fermentable fibres present, non-fermentable fibres like cellulose, among other factors. The presence or absence of these may be responsible for affecting the efficacy of drugs.

Dose and dosing regimen: This refers to the specific details of how a drug is administered to a patient, including the dose amount, frequency, and timing. Some key aspects of the dose and dosing regimen that can impact pharmacokinetics include:

- ***Dose amount***: This refers to type and quality of drug administered per dose that may affect the peak concentration and total exposure.
- ***Dosing frequency***: This focuses on how often the drug is given (such as once daily, twice daily), which impacts the duration of time the drug will course.
- ***Route of administration***: This focuses on the path by which the drug enters the body (e.g., oral, intravenous), that influences absorption.
- ***Dosing duration***: This focuses on the time during which the drug is administered, which is much relevant for chronic conditions.

However, it is also most relevant to know that the dosing regimen may need to be adjusted to suit a patient's conditions based on patient factors that alter pharmacokinetics. Some of these factors are:

- ***Renal or hepatic impairment***: Reduced activity requires dose alterations (usually a reduction or less frequent intake).
- ***Age***: In paediatric or geriatric populations there is a requirement for appropriate regimens that focus on altered ADME.
- ***Drug interactions***: Naturally accommodating medications that can induce or inhibit drug-metabolizing enzymes impact dosing.

10.1.2 DRUG DISTRIBUTION

Distribution refers to the movement of a drug from the bloodstream into various tissues, organs, and fluids of the body. It occurs after absorption and before metabolism and is responsible for the determination of where drugs will exert their effect within the body.

Distribution is important as it not only highlights the movement of the drug but also informs clinicians on the regimen to deploy based on presentations after interaction with the drugs administered.

For the context of our education, we would like to focus on a few thematic areas that augment and facilitate understanding of how distribution occurs in the pharmacokinetics of parasitic diseases or infections.

- Tissue distribution: Drug distribution to different tissues and organs in the body may have a significant impact on the therapeutic effect and potential side effects.
- In that, drugs that are well distributed to their target tissues or organs are more likely to achieve desired pharmacological results.
- Drugs with a high accumulation in non-target tissues may lead to unwanted side effects such as nephrotoxicity, neurotoxicity, hepatotoxicity, and cardiotoxicity, just to name a few.
- Sometimes, the size and physicochemical properties of drug molecules can influence tissue distribution. This is explained in an earlier chapter (Physiology and Biochemistry of Parasites – under types of transport). Smaller molecules tend to have better tissue penetration, whereas larger molecules tend to have little success compared to their smaller partners.
- We could also consider the binding of drugs to plasma proteins, such as the human serum albumin, that can affect the distribution of drugs by limiting their ability to reach target tissues.
- Pharmacokinetic–pharmacodynamic relationship: Also known as the PK–PD relationship. It describes the link between the drug concentrations at the site of action and the resulting pharmacological effect. In that regard:
- Drugs that result in higher concentrations at the target site are more likely to elicit a stronger pharmacological response. This explains why the most extreme pain reliefs are prescribed to people in dire need of relief (an example being morphine administered to sickle cell patients in a crisis).

- The time course of drug distribution to the target site can influence onset, duration, and the intensity of the drug's effect.
- Understanding the PK–PD relationship is essential for optimizing the drug dose and regimen to achieve the desired therapeutic effect while reducing adverse effects.

10.1.2.1 Factors that Influence Drug Distribution

Some other key factors that influence the distribution of drugs include:

- ***Volume of distribution (Vd)***: A parameter that represents the theoretical volume in which the total amount of drug would need to be uniformly distributed to give the observed blood concentration. An increased Vd shows extensive distribution into tissues and a decrease in Vd shows the drugs remain primarily in the bloodstream. It is worth noting that it varies among antiparasitic drugs.
- ***Protein binding***: Protein binding greatly affects drug distribution. Many drugs bind to plasma proteins (e.g., albumin). An example is praziquantel, which is highly protein-bound.
- Some drugs, like ivermectin, distribute widely into tissues.

10.1.3 DRUG METABOLISM

Metabolism is the biochemical process by which the body chemically alters drugs, usually through enzymatic systems mainly in the liver, to facilitate their elimination. This process often transforms drugs into more water-soluble compounds called metabolites, which can be inactive, active, or sometimes toxic.

Metabolism influences the duration and intensity of a drug's effects and plays a critical role in drug clearance from the body. It is an integral portion of the ADME process as it also oversees the overall disposition of a drug and can significantly influence the therapeutic properties of the drug while ensuring a safety profile. Drug metabolism also references the biochemical modifications that constitute a drug's makeup, usually in the liver, to make it more water-soluble and easier to excrete. The host of main enzymes usually involved in drug metabolism are:

- ***Cytochrome P450 enzyme (CYPs)***: These enzymes are responsible for Phase I metabolism, which includes redox reactions or hydrolysis of the drug molecule. For instance, albendazole is converted to its active metabolite, albendazole sulphoxide, by liver enzymes.
- ***Conjugation enzymes***: As the name infers, they are enzymes present in Phase II metabolism that conjugate with endogenous molecules like glucuronic acid, sulphate or glutathione to increase polarity.

The above are not the only contributing enzymes or factors that influence metabolism. Some other factors include:

- Genetic polymorphisms in metabolic enzymes.
- Age (elders usually having a reduced metabolism, which is only natural).
- Disease states depend on the affected organ and its implications, e.g., liver or kidney disease.
- Drug interactions (do they inhibit or induce metabolic enzymes?).
- Route of administration (e.g., first-pass metabolism after oral dosing).

The metabolites formed during drug metabolism can have various effects, including but not limited to:

- Some metabolites are inactive and simply facilitate the elimination of the drug.
- Other metabolites may be pharmacologically active and contribute to the overall therapeutic effect or toxicity of the drug.
- In some cases, metabolites can be more potent or have a different pharmacological profile compared to the parent drug.

PS: Many antiparasitic drugs undergo hepatic metabolism.

10.1.4 DRUG EXCRETION

Drug excretion is the process by which drugs and their metabolites are removed from the body, marking the final stage of pharmacokinetics after absorption, distribution, and metabolism. Efficient excretion is essential to terminate drug action and prevent accumulation that could lead to toxicity.

The kidneys serve as the principal organs of drug excretion, primarily eliminating water-soluble substances through urine. Drug elimination via the kidneys involves three main mechanisms: Glomerular filtration, active tubular secretion, and passive tubular reabsorption. Only unbound (free) drug molecules in plasma are filtered through the glomerulus. In the renal tubules, drugs may be actively secreted into the urine or reabsorbed back into the bloodstream depending on their ionic state, lipid solubility, and urine pH. Besides the kidneys, other important routes include:

- Biliary excretion, where the liver secretes drug metabolites into bile that enter the gastrointestinal tract and are eliminated in faeces.
- Pulmonary excretion, where gases and volatile substances like anaesthetic gases and alcohol are expelled via the lungs.
- Minor routes such as saliva, perspiration, tears, and breast milk also contribute to drug elimination but to a lesser extent.

The rate and extent of drug excretion can be influenced by factors such as kidney function (measured by glomerular filtration rate and creatinine clearance), age, biological sex, and drug interactions. For example, acidic or basic drugs can have their excretion altered by urine pH manipulation, a concept exploited in poisoning treatments to enhance elimination via "ion trapping."

Drug excretion is closely linked with metabolism since many hydrophobic drugs undergo biotransformation in the liver to more hydrophilic metabolites that are readily excreted by the kidneys. Hepatic metabolism occurs in two phases: Phase I modifies the drug molecule (oxidation, reduction, hydrolysis, often via cytochrome P450 enzymes), and Phase II conjugates the drug to polar molecules, enhancing solubility. Enzyme induction or inhibition (notably of CYP3A4) can markedly affect drug metabolism and subsequent excretion, altering plasma concentrations and risk of toxicity.

10.2 PHARMACOKINETIC PARAMETERS

These parameters provide a quantitative measurement of drug behaviour in the body. They include bioavailability, clearance, volume of distribution, and half-life.

- ***Bioavailability***: It describes the fraction of an administered dose that reaches systemic circulation and is available for action.
- ***Half-life (t1/2)***: Varies widely. For example, praziquantel has a short half-life of 1–3 hours, while ivermectin's half-life is about 18 hours.
- ***Clearance***: Reflects how quickly the drug is removed from the body, emphasizing both metabolism and excretion.
- ***Volume of distribution***: This describes the obvious space in the body where a drug is distributed, relative to the drug's concentration in the plasma.

10.3 SPECIAL CONSIDERATIONS IN PARASITOLOGY

The issue of special cases rides true even in the field of pharmacokinetics relative to parasitological infections. Some of these considerations include:

- ***Tissue penetration***: Some parasites reside in difficult-to-reach areas. For example, drugs treating neurocysticercosis must cross the blood–brain barrier.
- ***Intracellular activity***: Drugs treating intracellular parasites (e.g., *Leishmania*) must penetrate host cells.
- ***Life cycle stages***: Different parasite life stages may require different drug concentrations or treatment durations.
- ***Drug resistance***: Some parasites develop resistance mechanisms affecting drug uptake or efflux, impacting effective concentrations.

10.4 CURRENT ANTIPARASITIC DRUG TARGETS

The fight against parasitic infections continues to rage. These tiny invaders disproportionately affect vulnerable populations. Antiparasitic drugs aim to weaken parasites through targeted attacks.

Enzyme inhibition: Targeting essential enzymes is a common and potent strategy for inhibiting parasites. For example, drugs like primaquine starve malaria parasites by targeting enzymes involved in haemoglobin digestion. Similarly, metronidazole disrupts DNA synthesis in trichomonads, preventing replication.

Microtubule disruption: Microtubules, crucial for cell division and movement, are an appealing target. Benzimidazoles, used against helminths and protozoa, interfere with microtubule assembly, impeding parasite growth and motility. Ivermectin, a versatile drug, binds to parasite tubulin, immobilizing the organism and making it susceptible to the host's immune system.

Membrane disruption: The parasite's cell membrane is vulnerable to disruption by antifungal drugs. Amphotericin B disrupts the membrane, causing cell death. Praziquantel disrupts calcium homeostasis in schistosomes, leading to expulsion due to muscle spasms.

Signal blockade: Anthelmintics like levamisole bind to parasite nicotinic acetylcholine receptors, paralysing their neuromuscular system and rendering them unable to feed or reproduce. Miltefosine, a drug effective against leishmaniasis, disrupts parasite signalling pathways involved in cell division and differentiation, effectively halting their growth and replication.

Immune system boosters: While most antiparasitic drugs directly target the parasite, some work by enhancing the host's immune response. Interferon-alpha stimulates natural killer cells, bolstering the body's defences against viral parasites like hepatitis C. Additionally, praziquantel's immunemodulatory effects contribute to its potent action against schistosomes. Resistance to drugs endangers the effectiveness of previously effective drugs. In response, scientists are constantly creating new drug combinations and investigating new targets.

Combination therapy: Utilizing different drugs can delay resistance and improve effectiveness. ACTs are now the primary treatment for malaria, using multiple drugs to fight resistant strains.

Novel targets: Investigating unexplored pathways, such as lipid biosynthesis and protein translation, shows great potential. New drugs targeting these pathways are being developed, providing hope for reduced drug resistance in the future.

The future of antiparasitic drugs goes beyond targeting isolated cellular processes. There is a change towards holistic approaches that consider the interaction between the parasite, the host, and the environment.

Vaccines: Developing effective vaccines against key parasites, like malaria and schistosomiasis, would revolutionize prevention efforts. Ongoing research and promising clinical trials offer a glimmer of hope for a future where prevention takes centre stage.

Gene editing: The emergence of CRISPR-Cas9 technology opens doors for targeted gene editing in parasites, potentially rendering them sterile or susceptible to existing drugs. While ethical considerations and technical hurdles remain, the potential of this technology is undeniable.

Immunomodulation: Boosting the host's natural defences against parasites, through personalized immune response modulation, offers a promising avenue for tackling chronic and difficult-to-treat infections.

10.5 EXAMPLES OF ANTIPARASITIC DRUG PHARMACOKINETICS

To combat parasitic infections, the use of drugs, be they oral or otherwise, must be employed beyond the prevention phase. Some drugs that have been of importance across the years are as follows:

- Albendazole:
  - Poorly absorbed orally; fatty meals increase absorption.
  - Rapidly metabolized to active albendazole sulphoxide.
  - Half-life of active metabolite: 8–12 hours.
- Ivermectin:
  - Oral bioavailability: ~60%.
  - Widely distributed in tissues.
  - Long half-life allows for single-dose treatments in many cases.
- Praziquantel:
  - Rapidly absorbed orally.
  - Extensively metabolized in the liver.
  - Short half-life necessitates multiple doses in some treatments.

10.5.1 IMPLICATIONS FOR TREATMENT

As with all drugs, there is the need for precautions. Although there is alleviation of pain, there is also the possibility of side effects or other complications based on allergies and similar cases. Some implications to consider when tackling the issue of treatment are:

- Dosing schedules are based on pharmacokinetic properties.
- Drug–drug interactions can affect antiparasitic efficacy.
- Patient factors (e.g., age, liver/kidney function) may necessitate dose adjustments.

Finally, understanding the pharmacokinetics of antiparasitic drugs is essential for many reasons. To begin with, it aids in effective treatment and guides dosing strategies. It also helps predict drug efficacy and toxicity. It informs the development of new antiparasitic agents. As parasites continue to evolve resistance mechanisms, improved and increased funding, mass education and ongoing research in this field remain crucial as means of tackling the infection rates among other complications that it presents.

10.6 HERBAL MEDICINE IN THE TREATMENT OF PARASITIC DISEASES

Parasitic diseases, caused by organisms such as protozoa, helminths, and ectoparasites, continue to pose significant health challenges worldwide, particularly in regions with limited access to modern pharmaceuticals. Throughout history, herbal medicine has played a crucial role in the prevention and management of these diseases. The use of plant-based remedies is deeply rooted in traditional medical systems and remains an important therapeutic option in many communities today.

10.6.1 COMMON MEDICINAL PLANTS WITH ANTIPARASITIC PROPERTIES

A wide variety of medicinal plants have been employed in the treatment of parasitic infections. Scientific studies have begun to validate the effectiveness of many traditional remedies, highlighting the potential of herbal medicine as a complementary or alternative approach. Some of the most notable plants include:

- ***Neem (Azadirachta indica)***: Known for its broad-spectrum antiparasitic activity, neem is particularly effective against gastrointestinal nematodes. Its bioactive compounds disrupt the life cycle of parasites and enhance the host's immune response.
- ***Garlic (Allium sativum)***: Garlic contains sulphur-rich compounds that exhibit activity against a range of parasites,

including protozoa and helminths. It has been traditionally used to expel intestinal worms and treat protozoal infections.

- ***Wormwood (Artemisia absinthium)***: This plant has a long history of use against intestinal worms. Its active constituents, such as artemisinin, are also the basis for modern antimalarial therapies.
- ***Thyme (Thymus vulgaris)***: The essential oils in thyme have demonstrated efficacy against roundworms, tapeworms, and protozoa in laboratory studies.
- ***Ginger (Zingiber officinale)***: Traditionally used for amoebiasis and other parasitic infections, ginger's essential oils contribute to its antiparasitic effects.
- ***Oregano (Origanum vulgare)***: Oregano extracts and essential oils have shown promise against parasites responsible for diseases such as toxoplasmosis and giardiasis.

10.6.2 PREPARATION AND ADMINISTRATION

Herbal remedies are prepared and administered in various forms, including:

- **Decoctions and infusions** (herbal teas)
- **Extracts** (methanolic, ethanolic, or aqueous)
- Powders
- Essential oils

The preparation method and dosage often depend on the specific plant, the type of parasite, and the patient's condition.

10.6.3 MECHANISMS OF ACTION

The antiparasitic effects of medicinal plants are attributed to their rich content of bioactive compounds, such as alkaloids, flavonoids, terpenoids, and essential oils. These substances may:

- Disrupt parasite metabolism or reproduction.
- Exhibit direct toxic effects on parasites.
- Modulate the host's immune system to enhance resistance.

10.6.4 SCIENTIFIC EVIDENCE AND EFFICACY

A growing body of research supports the antiparasitic activity of many medicinal plants. For instance, methanolic extracts of *Chiranthodendron pentadactylon* and *Annona cherimola* have demonstrated activity against *Entamoeba histolytica*. Essential oils from mint, clove, and thyme have shown efficacy against gastrointestinal parasites in laboratory studies. Moreover, combinations of plant extracts may offer enhanced therapeutic effects compared to single extracts.

Despite these promising findings, most evidence is derived from laboratory and animal studies. Comprehensive clinical trials in human populations are still limited, underscoring the need for further research.

10.6.5 SAFETY CONSIDERATIONS

While herbal medicines offer valuable alternatives, several important considerations must be addressed:

- ***Standardization***: The lack of standardized dosages and preparation methods can affect both safety and efficacy.
- ***Side effects and interactions***: Some herbs may cause adverse effects or interact with conventional medications.
- ***Regulation***: Herbal supplements are often subject to less rigorous regulatory oversight compared to pharmaceutical drugs.

Herbal medicine remains a vital resource in the management of parasitic diseases, particularly in resource-limited settings. Plants such as neem, garlic, wormwood, thyme, and ginger have demonstrated significant antiparasitic properties, supported by both traditional use and scientific research. However, to fully realize the potential of herbal remedies, further studies – including well-designed clinical trials – are essential to establish standardized protocols, safety profiles, and efficacy in human populations.

10.7 DEFINITIONS

Bioavailability *refers to the degree and rate at which a drug or substance is absorbed and becomes available at the site of action in the body.*

Absorption rate *refers to the speed at which a drug or substance is absorbed from the site of administration into the systemic circulation.*

FURTHER READING

https://www.ncbi.nlm.nih.gov/books/NBK557405/
https://edu.rsc.org/download?ac=12812#:~:text=Active%20transport%20is%20when%20a,its%20concentration%20is%20already%20higher
https://www.youtube.com/watch?v=BfPx-DnZIDA
https://pubmed.ncbi.nlm.nih.gov/21956605/
https://www.ncbi.nlm.nih.gov/pmc/articles/PMC9311319/
https://pubmed.ncbi.nlm.nih.gov/23227553/
https://www.ncbi.nlm.nih.gov/pmc/articles/PMC8635734/
https://www.ncbi.nlm.nih.gov/pmc/articles/PMC9311319/
https://www.semanticscholar.org/paper/1b5372738eb7b8ce2b6257b1a863794bb5b39e70
https://www.ncbi.nlm.nih.gov/pmc/articles/PMC10197202/
https://www.longdom.org/open-access/the-pharmacokinetic-parameters-and-significance-in-medicine-101474.html#:~:text=Pharmacokinetic%20parameters%20provide%20quantitative%20measurements,and%20is%20available%20for%20action

Index

For Product Safety Concerns and Information please contact our EU
representative GPSR@taylorandfrancis.com
Taylor & Francis Verlag GmbH, Kaufingerstraße 24, 80331 München, Germany

www.ingramcontent.com/pod-product-compliance
Lightning Source LLC
LaVergne TN
LVHW021416220826
846195LV00027B/246

* 9 7 8 1 0 4 1 2 2 3 9 8 6 *